Thanks for all your support in the cafe. We look forward to a great 2009. Chef Hugo (Mike)

The Inner Peace Diet

by
**Aileen McCabe-Maucher
and Hugo Maucher**

ALPHA

A member of Penguin Group (USA) Inc.

This book is dedicated to our daughter, Vivian, our source of divine inspiration. We love you unconditionally and without limits for all of eternity. Always remember that you are connected to inner peace and all living things in every moment.

ALPHA BOOKS

Published by the Penguin Group

Penguin Group (USA) Inc., 375 Hudson Street, New York, New York 10014, USA

Penguin Group (Canada), 90 Eglinton Avenue East, Suite 700, Toronto, Ontario M4P 2Y3, Canada (a division of Pearson Penguin Canada Inc.)

Penguin Books Ltd., 80 Strand, London WC2R 0RL, England

Penguin Ireland, 25 St. Stephen's Green, Dublin 2, Ireland (a division of Penguin Books Ltd.)

Penguin Group (Australia), 250 Camberwell Road, Camberwell, Victoria 3124, Australia (a division of Pearson Australia Group Pty. Ltd.)

Penguin Books India Pvt. Ltd., 11 Community Centre, Panchsheel Park, New Delhi—110 017, India

Penguin Group (NZ), 67 Apollo Drive, Rosedale, North Shore, Auckland 1311, New Zealand (a division of Pearson New Zealand Ltd.)

Penguin Books (South Africa) (Pty.) Ltd., 24 Sturdee Avenue, Rosebank, Johannesburg 2196, South Africa

Penguin Books Ltd., Registered Offices: 80 Strand, London WC2R 0RL, England

International Standard Book Number: 978-1-59257-815-3

Library of Congress Catalog Card Number: 2008929017

10 09 08   8 7 6 5 4 3 2 1

Interpretation of the printing code: The rightmost number of the first series of numbers is the year of the book's printing; the rightmost number of the second series of numbers is the number of the book's printing. For example, a printing code of 08-1 shows that the first printing occurred in 2008.

Printed in the United States of America

Note: This publication contains the opinions and ideas of its authors. It is intended to provide helpful and informative material on the subject matter covered. It is sold with the understanding that the authors and publisher are not engaged in rendering professional services in the book. If the reader requires personal assistance or advice, a competent professional should be consulted.

The authors and publisher specifically disclaim any responsibility for any liability, loss, or risk, personal or otherwise, which is incurred as a consequence, directly or indirectly, of the use and application of any of the contents of this book.

Most Alpha books are available at special quantity discounts for bulk purchases for sales promotions, premiums, fund-raising, or educational use. Special books, or book excerpts, can also be created to fit specific needs.

For details, write: Special Markets, Alpha Books, 375 Hudson Street, New York, NY 10014.

Publisher: *Marie Butler-Knight*
Editorial Director: *Mike Sanders*
Senior Managing Editor: *Billy Fields*
Development Editor: *Ginny Bess Munroe*
Production Editor: *Megan Douglass*
Copy Editor: *Jan Zoya*
Cover/Book Designer: *Kurt Owens*
Indexer: *Heather McNeill*
Layout: *Ayanna Lacey*
Proofreader: *Laura Caddell*

Contents

Introduction

Are you looking for a way to lose weight and eliminate stress from your life? You hold in your hands the answer you have been seeking. *The Inner Peace Diet* is a revolutionary book that will help you lose weight and live the life of your dreams. This book differs from many other diet and self-help books on the shelf because it is not strictly about theory. It is about honoring yourself. This extraordinary diet was created by a registered nurse, licensed psychotherapist, and acclaimed master chef. By implementing this innovative seven-week plan, you will shed unwanted pounds and gain a sense of eternal serenity. The Inner Peace Diet will transform your body and mind so that you can attain the permanent joy and tranquility you are in search of. Through following the guidelines in this unique book, you will obtain not only your ideal body but your ideal life.

In today's world, grocery stores shelves are overflowing with beautifully packaged convenience food that can be prepared in a matter of seconds. As a working parent, I am sometimes tempted to make a highly processed or frozen meal because it just seems faster and easier. Although these convenience items save us time today, consuming these foods may put our long-term health and well-being in jeopardy. The trouble is, most processed foods are laden with trans fat, refined sugar, high fructose corn syrup, food coloring, and other preservatives. Some food additives have been linked to diseases such as atherosclerosis, diabetes, and attention deficit disorder. Attempt to eat as many fresh fruits and vegetables as you can, and strive to eat food that comes from Mother Nature instead of a box. Eat foods that are in season locally, instead of purchasing the canned or frozen varieties. Instead of devouring foods laden with white flour and sugar, infuse your diet with whole grains and use natural sweeteners like honey or fruit. Read nutritional labels and do not consume foods that contain high fructose corn syrup, trans fat, refined sugar, or dyes. It is also helpful to limit your consumption of dairy products and animal products that are high in fat.

Best-selling author and physician Deepak Chopra stresses the importance of a healthy chakra system in his books and workshops. The ancient science of yoga is focused entirely on balancing the chakra system and is currently practiced by 30 million people worldwide. The holistic Indian practice of Ayurveda has been practiced for five thousand years and centers on the chakras. Lisa Oz, wife of Mehment Oz, M.D. who is co-author of the best-selling *YOU on a Diet* series, concentrates on the importance of the chakra system in her life's work as a Reiki Master, author, and speaker.

About Your Chakra System

Each chakra represents a spectrum of vibrating electrical energy through which we process life experiences and emotions. Ideally, all seven chakras will emit the same amount of energy. When functioning properly, the chakras spin like whirlpools in a clockwise direction as they regulate our energies, emotions, and health. If this energy is blocked, physical and/or psychiatric illness will manifest.

The lowest chakra corresponds to our fundamental survival needs such as food and shelter. As the chakras move up the body, they relate to our higher level needs such as communication and spirituality. The first chakra is located in the genitals and is called the root chakra. This energy center is associated with the color red and the adrenal glands. The second chakra is known as the sacral chakra and is located in the uterus in women and the spleen in men. This chakra is represented by the color orange. The third chakra is called the solar plexus and is located near the lower ribs and associated with the color yellow. Diseases associated with an unbalanced solar plexus include alcoholism, eating disorders, and digestive problems. Above the solar plexus is the fourth chakra, otherwise known as the heart chakra. The heart chakra is behind the sternum and physically associated with the thymus gland and the heart. The fifth, throat chakra is located at the base of the neck and associated with the color blue. The throat chakra is associated with the thyroid and parathyroid glands, and creativity and emotions are expressed through this energy center. The sixth chakra is known as the brow or third-eye chakra and is located above and between the eyes. Associated with the pituitary gland, this chakra is also known as an individual's intuition center and is often paired with the colors indigo and violet. The final and seventh chakra is the crown chakra, located at the top of the head behind the skull. This chakra is physically associated with the pineal gland and represents a person's connection with their spirituality and with the universe. The crown chakra is usually represented by the colors violet and white.

The seven chakras form a holistic organism; they all must be in order for a person to be in harmony with the world and reach their full potential. The chakra system is best described as an internal rainbow through which we can acheive inner peace and attain our greatest desires.

The most common symptoms of unbalanced and blocked chakras are weight gain and obesity. Please do not use this book as a tool to diagnose yourself or others. If you are obese or experiencing physical or psychological problems, we urge you to seek the guidance of a licensed, credentialed health expert. For in-depth information about your chakra system, I highly recommend that you read *Anatomy of the Spirit* by Caroline Myss, Ph.D.

This book is designed to balance the chakras, promote weight loss, and create a sense of lasting peace and contentment. The Inner Peace Diet is a seven-week eating plan featuring easy-to-prepare delicious recipes created by a master chef. All the ingredients can be purchased at your local grocery store and most of the entrees can be prepared in less than thirty minutes. Each week focuses on specific foods that will enhance that chakra's optimal functioning. This book encourages eating fresh, organic fruits and vegetables. Research has consistently shown that eating a variety of rainbow-colored vegetables containing phytonutrients promotes longevity and wards off cancer and heart disease.

How the Book is Organized

This book is divided into eight easy-to-read chapters. The chapters focus on each of the major chakra systems in the body, chakras one through seven, respectively. The final chapter focuses on combining healthy foods representing all of the chakras and maintaining a healthy lifestyle and weight throughout your time on Earth. Each chapter contains at least three breakfast recipes, three lunch recipes, four dinner recipes, two dessert recipes, and a host of healthy snacks. A comprehensive list of chakra-enhancing foods and spices is included in each chapter. In addition to the easy-to-follow eating plan, each chapter features exercises that focus on psychological and emotional healing. These exercises are designed to help you achieve a sense of self-mastery, fulfillment, and inner peace and can readily be incorporated into a busy, fast-paced lifestyle.

Created by a licensed psychotherapist who has helped many people lose weight, these techniques will help you attain a level of happiness greater than you ever imagined. These proven self-help methods combine cognitive behavioral therapy, self-hypnosis, and Gestalt therapy with ancient spiritual traditions. Some exercises are illustrated by examples that clearly demonstrate how real clients' lives have been transformed by these techniques. Some chapters include meditations that can be used each day to reinforce new eating behaviors. This book is appropriate for people of all religious backgrounds and traditions and encourages people to be who they are.

Chapter One, "Your Root Chakra"

The root chakra corresponds to your fundamental survival needs, such as food and shelter. Located in the genitals, the first chakra reflects your ability to feel safe and secure in this world. This energy center is associated with the color red and the adrenal glands. This chapter features 19 gourmet recipes that contain root-chakra-enhancing whole foods. Additionally, this chapter includes seven personal-growth exercises that will increase your sense of security.

Chapter Two, "Your Sacral Chakra"

The second chakra is known as the sacral chakra. It is located in the uterus in women and the spleen in men. This chakra is represented by the color orange, and it reflects a person's ability to seek pleasure in life. Chapter two contains 16 healthy, easy-to-prepare recipes. Furthermore, this chapter includes nine self-help exercises designed to help you attain pleasure and get in touch with your emotions.

Chapter Three, "Your Solar Plexus Chakra"

Associated with the concepts of identity and self-esteem, the third chakra is housed near the lower ribs, and is represented by the color yellow. Twenty-two nutritious recipes are featured in this chapter of the book. This chapter features 10 personal-growth exercises that will help you get a clear sense of your life's purpose and break free of procrastination and powerlessness.

Chapter Four, "Your Heart Chakra"

The heart chakra is physically associated with the chest cavity and the color green. This chakra reflects your ability to give and receive love and compassion. Eighteen heart-opening, heart-healthy recipes are featured in this chapter. Seven personal-growth exercises will help you experience true compassion, love, and devotion toward yourself and others.

Chapter Five, "Your Throat Chakra"

The throat chakra is physically located near the neck, and is represented by the color blue. A thriving throat chakra enables you to connect with yourself and others in a deep and satisfying way. This chapter is comprised of 16 healthy recipes designed to bring your throat chakra into balance. Additionally, eight personal-growth exercises will help you communicate more effectively with others and speak your truth.

Chapter Six, "Your Third-Eye Chakra"

The sixth chakra is associated with the color purple, and is linked with both physical and intuitive vision. Physically, the third-eye chakra is located between the eyebrows. This chapter offers 17 third-eye chakra-enhancing gourmet recipes. Also included in this chapter are 10 personal-growth exercises that will help you develop your ability to trust in your inner wisdom and intuitive powers.

Chapter Seven, "Your Crown Chakra"

The seventh chakra represents spiritual enlightenment and union with the sacred and all living things. This chakra is located on top of the head, and is represented by the color white. This chapter includes 18 gourmet recipes, many of which are ethnic dishes that celebrate diversity. We also give you 10 self-help exercises to help you create an enhanced sense of spiritual consciousness and fulfill your destiny.

Chapter Eight, "Your Entire Chakra System: The Rainbow Within"

The final chapter summarizes the function of all seven chakras, and emphasizes the importance of maintaining a healthy, balanced lifestyle. This chapter features 11 recipes that will integrate food from all of the preceding seven chapters. By focusing on a combination of mind, body, and spirit techniques, this chapter will reinforce the new behaviors and concepts you learned in the book. Additionally, this chapter contains a meditation exercise, and teaches you how to draw on your inner wisdom to maintain your newfound weight loss and serenity.

Although the Inner Peace Diet will help you lose pounds quickly and effortlessly, it is not a fad diet. Rather it is a lifelong plan that encourages you to eat healthy foods and to feed your mind and soul with joyful thoughts. In order to attain permanent weight loss you must change your eating habits in conjunction with your thoughts and behavior. Each day you are invited to take seven steps that will virtually guarantee permanent weight loss and inner bliss. The number seven is considered to be a sacred and lucky number in most of the world's spiritual and religious traditions. It is a number that represents wisdom and growth, and was considered to be a perfect number by Pygathoras and ancient Chinese scholars. Following are the seven steps you need to take each day to begin your journey to permanent weight loss and inner peace:

- Meditate
- Keep a Journal

- Exercise
- Set your intention for the day
- Make a daily gratitude list
- Incorporate live, organic foods into your diet
- Visualize your ideal body and lifestyle

Meditate for a Happy and Healthier Life

Meditation grounds the first chakra and also helps all seven chakras function optimally. It is one of the best-kept secrets to a fit body, mind, and soul. Additionally, it is a vital component to inner peace and permanent weight loss. People who meditate daily report feeling a sense of greater serenity and purpose. In addition, many people find that meditation can help them achieve their weight-loss goals and dramatically reduce life's stressors. Learning to meditate can be a challenging process. However, once you get the hang of it, meditation will likely be your favorite part of the day.

Meditation is best defined as a time of inner reflection. With practice, you will experience a vast sense of peace and contentment during your meditation time. Meditation is the best way to nourish your soul and give your mind the rest it craves. It quiets the endless chatter and dialogue that is constantly going on in your head. When you first start to meditate you may find yourself drifting off to sleep or having a hard time sitting still. These feelings of sleepiness and restlessness are completely normal. Trust your individual experience and know that you are making progress.

It is best to meditate twice a day, once in the morning and once in the evening. Each meditation session should be at least twenty minutes in duration. In today's busy and fast-paced world it can be difficult to find forty extra minutes each day. If you are short on time, resist the temptation to skip this exercise. Begin your practice by setting aside a mere five minutes each day to meditate. Start from where you are and what feels comfortable to you. As your meditation skills improve and you reap the rewards of daily practice, you will want to devote more time to inner reflection.

Choose a meditation space where you will not be interrupted. This place should be away from distractions such as the telephone, computer, and doorbell. Look around your home for a place that feels quiet and inviting. Ideally this area will be free of clutter and should not be associated with stressful triggers such as work problems or traumatic events. It is important for you to be able to feel as relaxed as possible when you enter your meditative process. Many people choose to meditate outside in nature. For others the only quiet place they can access is their bathroom. You may want to create a meditation table or altar to inspire you. Your meditation altar can include pictures of loved ones, statues, religious relics, or other treasured items to enhance your time of inner reflection. There is no right or wrong place to meditate and become one with your spirit.

There are many different types of meditation. Some meditations involve the use of mantras or repeated words or phrases. Other meditations encourage you to visualize various images in your mind's eye. Walking meditations are yet another way to bask in a sense of limitless peace. Each chapter in this book will feature a different meditation technique. Experiment with all the various techniques and decide for yourself which one works best for you.

A Simple Introductory Meditation

We recommend that you dictate this meditation, as well as all of the other meditations in the book, into a voice recorder. When you are ready to meditate, simply play the recordings and follow the instructions. After a few weeks of practice, you will probably find that you no longer need to hear a recording of the meditation and will be able to achieve this state of being on your own.

Sit on the floor or on a pillow with your legs crossed. Alternatively, you can sit on a chair with both feet placed firmly on the floor. Keep your back straight and envision each vertebra stacking one on top of the other, bone by bone. Place your hands on your knees with your palms facing up. You may choose to keep your eyes open, gazing past the tip of your nose or you can meditate with your eyes closed.

As you begin your meditation say aloud or to yourself "I am totally relaxed, surrounded by peace and love."

State your intention for this meditation. Choose an objective that feels right for you and meets your needs on that particular day. Some examples of intentions are "I dedicate this meditation to creating a healthy body." "I devote this meditation to world peace." "During this meditation, I intend to let go of negative feelings and replace them with peace and joy."

Focus on your breathing. Slowly breathe in and out through your nostrils. Allow your whole body to relax. Let go of any muscle tension or anxiety. Gently let go of any stressful thoughts or worries.

Visualize a blank television screen in your mind's eye. Allow all of your thoughts to disappear. When your mind starts forming thoughts, words, or pictures gently notice these thought forms. Then, bring your focus back to the blank television screen.

Focus on your breathing and bodily sensations, without trying to engage them. If you are feeling tired or restless, notice these feelings and sensations and give yourself permission to experience them. Do not resist or judge anything that arises. Focus on breathing in and out and allowing everything to be as it is in this moment.

If you are distracted by outside noises such as sirens, telephones, or rain, simply notice these distractions and let them go. Having thoughts occur during meditation is as natural as breathing. Welcome the thoughts and then quietly let them go as you surrender to silence. Focus on breathing in and breathing out. Continue this practice for twenty minutes. You may choose to meditate for as long as you desire. At the end of the mediation session, take several long, deep breaths. Feel a sense of gratitude and appreciation for this time of inner reflection.

Journal Writing

We encourage you to keep a journal in an effort to lose weight and feel happy. Journal writing simply involves writing your thoughts, feelings, and experiences down on paper. Research indicates that people who express themselves through writing can boost their immune systems and decrease symptoms of certain illnesses, such as rheumatoid arthritis and asthma. You can choose to write your thoughts in your journal daily or just do the journal exercises contained in each chapter. This book contains numerous writing exercises that have lead many clients to a radical awakening of the mind, body, and spirit. Prior to beginning your diet, obtain a large notebook and pen. If you want, you can decorate your notebook with wrapping papers, artwork, or quotes that inspire you. Although writing in a journal can seem awkward or time-consuming at first, it is a great stress reliever and may soon become a favorite part of your day.

Exercise

Exercise is necessary to maintain a healthy body, mind, and spirit. It helps balance your chakra system and maintain other vital organ systems in your physical body. In order to keep your body functioning at an optimal level it is vital to keep it moving. Although, exercise may seem tedious or difficult at first, it can be a fun way to reconnect with yourself. When you exercise, potent chemicals in your brain called endorphins are released into your blood stream. These endorphins are similar to compounds used in prescription painkillers and antidepressants. Endorphin release stimulated by exercise generates feelings of intense relaxation and actually makes you want to engage in physical activity more frequently. Thus, exercise is a surefire way to change your mental state and increase inner peace. And it does not have to be a boring or lonely chore! While you are on this diet devote at least thirty minutes per day to physical fitness. Brisk walking, weightlifting, karate, and Pilates are all great ways to get into shape. Be adventurous and try a new fitness class or sport that interests you. Salsa dancing, kettle bells, krav maga, and belly dancing are all fun physical activities that can help you get fit and stay in shape. Yoga is a beneficial form of exercise that has been around for nearly two thousand years. This form of exercise helps align your chakras and increase strength and flexibility. Each chapter in *The Inner Peace Diet* features at least one yoga pose. Experiment with different forms of exercise to see which ones you enjoy.

Set Your Intention Each Day

Each day upon awakening, ask yourself, "What is my intention for the day?" This is really just another way of asking yourself "What do I want for myself and what am I willing to allow into my life?" Examples of daily intentions are "Today I intend to make healthy and nutritious food choices" or "My intention today is to extend kindness to every person that I encounter." Most people give very little thought to their daily desires. Chaotic, overscheduled lives often cause us to live in an unconscious way. As a result, we wind up creating lives that cause dissatisfaction and inner turmoil by default. Intention is a powerful tool that will help you manifest your heart's desire through the chakras. You may find that once you begin setting an intention each day, you feel the need to make drastic life changes related to your job, relationship status, or family life. Or perhaps the only things that will change is the way you view life and your newfound sense of joy. Declaring a daily intention will help you clarify your values and determine what will truly bring you happiness. In addition, your awareness will shift and you will attract the people, experiences, and things that you want into your life.

Incorporate Living, Organic Food into Your Diet Whenever Possible

In today's fast-paced world, commercially prepared convenience food is abundant. Although this prepackaged, highly processed food saves us time, it is at often great cost to our physical health. Processed foods typically contain fewer nutrients and are packed with preservatives and other questionable additives. Food that is laden in high fructose corn syrup, animal fat, trans fat, white flour, and refined sugar clogs our arteries, digestive systems, and our chakra centers. Many of these foods have addictive qualities and deplete our energy. Reduce or eliminate foods that contain red meat, refined flour, high fructose corn sugar, and high fat dairy. Strive to eat whole foods that are as close to their natural state as possible. Attempt to eat fresh fruits and vegetables whenever feasible, instead of purchasing frozen or canned products. Educate yourself about the food you eat and learn about how and where it is produced.

Make every effort to incorporate organic food into your diet as much as you can. Organic foods are grown or manufactured with little or no pesticides, hormones, antibiotics, or genetically modified ingredients. Due to increased consumer demand, most stores carry organic products. Although organic products are slightly more expensive than non-organic groceries, eating these foods may save you money on health-care expenses down the road. Try substituting the major staples on your grocery list for organic products. According to Dr. Alan Gleene, M.D., buying organic milk, eggs, apples, ketchup, and peanut butter are excellent ways to begin to eliminate pesticides from your diet. Typically these items are eaten in large quantities and produced in environments laden with additives. Studies show that organically grown foods may contain more antioxidants and nutrients and taste better than their non-organic counterparts. In addition, buying organic products helps protect the environment and sometimes helps put money back into your local economy.

Make a Daily Gratitude List

Each night before going to sleep, make a list of all the things that you are grateful for in your life. Learning to appreciate the things that you already have creates a tremendous sense of joy. Gratitude and appreciation align all seven of your major chakras and bring a sense of eternal peace to everyday living. As you author your nightly gratitude list, review your day and feel thankful for all the positive things that happened to you and helpful people that crossed your path. Some people find it useful to analyze the events of the day in sequential or reverse-chronological order. Remember that there is nothing too small or trivial to feel grateful about. Examples of items on a gratitude list include: "I am grateful for my daughter's beautiful smile." "I am so thankful for this bed I sleep in." or "I feel so grateful for the new toothbrush I used today." As you write your gratitude list, focus on the positive emotion that feeling thankful evokes within you. Even on the darkest of days, it is important that you attempt to complete this exercise. One suicidal client lamented that at times "I am grateful that I am breathing today" is the only item she could muster for her gratitude journal. When you feel as if you have completed your daily gratitude list, take a few moments and see if you can think of anything else to appreciate. It is also beneficial to fall asleep reciting your gratitude list silently to yourself. After just seven short weeks of keeping your gratitude journal, you will be amazed at all the new and exciting things you will have to be thankful for.

Visualize Your Ideal Body and Lifestyle

Spend at least five minutes each day envisioning your ideal body and lifestyle. Imagine exactly how you would look, feel, and carry yourself if you reached your goal weight. Make a list of all the things you want to be, do, or have. Review this list daily and imagine that all of these items have come to pass. Picture yourself as already living the life of your dreams. Visualization is a potent tool that uses the sixth chakra to bring desires into reality. Do not be concerned about how you will attain these things. This book contains many exercises that will assist you in how to create your ideal body and life.

Do This Exercise to Create Time on Your Clock

In today's society, many people are profoundly addicted to substances such as alcohol, drugs, or nicotine. Others are addicted to behaviors such as gambling, sex, or overeating. According to the American Heritage Dictionary, an addiction is defined as the condition of being habitually or compulsively occupied with or involved in something. Simply put, addictions destroy our root chakra's sense of connectedness to the earth. They are time-consuming practices that drain our energy and make us feel chronically insecure and anxious. When we experience an addiction of any kind, our sense of survival is annihilated. A person who in the throes of addiction spends the vast majority of his or her time focused on obtaining, using, or engaging in the negative behavior. Dependence upon powerful substances or self-destructive behaviors are typically complicated and life threatening. These are best managed with the help of a licensed professional. With proper treatment, addictions can be managed and serve as transformative life lessons. If you feel that you cannot stop using a substance or are consistently engaging in a self-destructive behavior, I urge you to seek help immediately. Your family doctor is a good place to start. Here are websites and phone numbers to help you on your journey to recovery.

- www.alcoholic-anonymous.org

- www.na.org

- The National Suicide Prevention Hotline 1-800-273-TALK

- National Child Abuse Hotline 1-800-4-A-CHILD

- National Domestic Violence Hotline 1-800-799-SAFE

Minor addictions to things such as e-mail and websurfing are also common in modern society. Although these behaviors are not life threatening, they often serve as crutches to alleviate anxiety. Paradoxically, these behaviors rob us of valuable time and prevent us from having the energy we need to pursue our dreams. Over the years, many clients have said to me, "I just don't have time to do these writing exercises and experiments that you recommend. I am way too busy." I completely understand the demands of life and empathize with their feelings. If you are feeling overwhelmed and starved for time I urge you to make a log of how you spend your time every day this week. Be vigilant in your analysis. Record every minute you spend listening to a friend complain, reading a junk e-mail, or aimlessly surfing the web. At the end of the week look at your time log. How do you spend the majority of your time? What are your "minor addictions"?

The first step to overcoming any addiction is acknowledging it. This week, make a list of the minor addictions that exist in your life. Popular minor addictions include: websurfing, watching television, chatting on the telephone, gossiping, worrying, creating endless to-do lists (and never implementing them), and spending time with negative people who drain your energy. After you have completed your list, sit quietly for ten minutes and visualize your life without these minor addictions. Then pick up your pen and prepare to take control of your life. Next to each minor addiction write a way that you can replace this undesired behavior with something positive. For example, while writing this book, I developed a pretty entrenched addiction to checking my e-mail. I knew things were out of control when I started sleeping with my blackberry and awakening every three hours to check my inbox. I decided that instead of checking my e-mail every twenty minutes, I would only read it twice a day. When I felt an overwhelming compulsion to scan my inbox at any other point during the day, I spent the ten minutes that I would have spent e-mailing, working on a scrapbook for my dad. Within days, I conquered my addiction and created a beautiful book for my terminally ill father. Most importantly, I felt the reemergence of a strong sense of security, accomplishment, and groundedness that had been missing during my minor e-mail addiction.

Things You Need to Do Before Starting the Diet

One week prior to beginning *The Inner Peace Diet*, keep a radically honest food diary. Obtain a small notebook and pen and carry it with you wherever you go. Record every single thing you put in your mouth for one entire week. Attempt to jot down any emotional triggers that are associated with eating. This exercise will help you become conscious about what you put in your mouth and your eating patterns.

Adequate amounts of sleep and rest are two vital components of a healthy lifestyle. Prior to beginning this diet, make every effort to get at least seven to nine hours sleep each night. It is also helpful if you can arrange to take a short twenty minute nap each afternoon. If napping seems impossible in your present circumstances, at least find a few minutes every day to put your head down and relax.

Prior to beginning this diet or any other diet, we recommend that you get a physical examination and discuss your individual nutritional needs with your doctor or health-care provider. Bring this book with you to your appointment and share it with your doctor. If you have a history of major depressive disorder, psychosis, or any significant mental health diagnosis, we recommend that you do these personal growth exercises under the guidance of a licensed, professional counselor. If you experience any feelings of depression that interfere with your daily life while you are reading this book or any other self-help title, I encourage you to seek the help of a licensed therapist. Your physician will likely approve of this healthy and sensible eating plan that is appropriate for just about anyone. Welcome to your new peaceful and healthy life!

Acknowledgments

We extend love and heartfelt gratitude to the following people:

Our mother, Colleen McCabe, for supporting our every endeavor with love and tireless childcare services.

Our mother, Mary Lou Maucher, for her love, support, and unyielding forthrightness.

Our father, John V. McCabe, for being a living example of unconditional love, true genius, and selfless service.

Our father, Hugo Robert Maucher, for his wisdom, love of food, and the human pursuit of happiness.

Our beloved family, especially grandmother Dolly McCabe, Uncle Eddie and Aunt Alma, Beth, The Patricks, Bill, Mary Beth, Bill, Katie, Ellen, Nancy, Gary, Chiara, Josef, Ani, Mary, Ema, and Kai.

Our yoga teacher, Dawn Mehan, for her divine wisdom.

Our agent, Stacey Glick, for her expert guidance and support.

Our acquisitions editor, Michele Wells, for her vision and direction, and for taking a huge chance on us. Our development editor, Ginny Bess Munroe, for her wisdom and guidance. Our copy editor, Jan Zoya, for her great advice and encouragement. Our editor Megan Douglass for her talent and exquisite attention to detail.

Our friends, whom we are so lucky to have in our lives! We wish that we you could name you all here. You are in our hearts forever.

Every living being in the universe, we wish you inner peace and joy!

Trademarks

All terms mentioned in this book that are known to be or are suspected of being trademarks or service marks have been appropriately capitalized. Alpha Books and Penguin Group (USA) Inc. cannot attest to the accuracy of this information. Use of a term in this book should not be regarded as affecting the validity of any trademark or service mark.

1

Your Root Chakra

Your first energy center is called the root chakra. Physically, it is located near your adrenal glands and genitals, deep within your pelvis. The root chakra is the lowest of the seven major chakras and is the energy center that sits closest to the ground. In order for you to be healthy, your first chakra must be firmly rooted to the earth. This energy center is represented by the color red, and is supported by wearing crimson hues.

Your first chakra directly reflects your ability to flourish in your environment. When you have a balanced and thriving root chakra, you enjoy feelings of safety, security, stability, and stillness.

If your root chakra is out of alignment, you may struggle to meet your basic survival needs. Financial difficulties, overwhelming debt, and employment troubles are the major signs of a dysfunctional first energy center.

When your first chakra is blocked, you feel uncomfortable in your own skin, and out of touch with your own bodily sensations and drives. Major life stressors such as job loss, divorce, addictions, pregnancy, or illness can trigger problems with the first chakra.

In order to stabilize the first chakra, you must establish a sense of being grounded and supported by the earth. After completing this week's eating plan and personal-growth exercises, you will feel grounded, secure, and connected to your body.

This week, reconnect to the earth by incorporating more fresh fruits and vegetables into your diet. Fruits and vegetables come from the earth and contain living, organic ingredients that help realign your root chakra to the earth. Your first chakra is also enhanced by eating lean proteins such as nuts, seeds, and lean meats. This week, focus on eliminating processed foods and eating only foods that are alive.

Let's start by getting your first chakra in balance by looking at the eating plan.

ROOT CHAKRA SEVEN-DAY EATING PLAN

Day One

Breakfast: Italian Egg-White Frittata
Midmorning Snack: 1 large Macintosh apple and ½ cup sunflower seeds
Lunch: Better Than Pizza Salad
Midafternoon Snack: ¼ cup walnuts
Dinner: Moroccan-Inspired Apple and Chicken Couscous
Dessert: Organic Strawberry Banana Cupcake

Day Two

Breakfast: Cottage Cheese Apple Pancakes
Midmorning Snack: ½ cup sliced strawberries
Lunch: Salmon-Infused Waldorf salad
Midafternoon Snack: ½ cup Chakra Salsa with celery and carrot sticks
Dinner: Tortilla Pie with Chakra Salsa
Dessert: Cherry Almond Oat Muffin

Day Three

Breakfast: Pomegranate Berry Smoothie
Midmorning Snack: ½ cup nonfat cottage cheese and 6 cherry tomatoes
Lunch: Strawberry Poppy Seed Salad
Midafternoon Snack: 1 slice watermelon
Dinner: Mike's Bean Salad with Red Peppers and Feta Cheese
Dessert: Sinful Baked Apples with Yogurt Sauce

Day Four

Breakfast: Cherry Almond Oat Muffin
Midmorning Snack: 1 large grapefruit
Lunch: Beet Soup with Carrots and Goat Cheese

Midafternoon Snack: 1/4 cup walnuts

Dinner: Cheesy Baked Chicken with Chakra Salsa

Dessert: Sweet and Sour Cherry Slaw

Day Five

Breakfast: Italian Egg-White Frittata

Midmorning Snack: 1/2 cup pumpkin seeds

Lunch: Root Vegetables Drenched in Honey

Midafternoon Snack: 1 large apple

Dinner: Whole-Wheat Vegetable Pita Pizza

Dessert: Organic Strawberry Banana Cupcake

Day Six

Breakfast: Cottage Cheese Apple Pancakes

Midmorning Snack: 1/2 cup dried cranberries

Lunch: Strawberry Poppy Seed Salad

Midafternoon Snack: 1/4 cup walnuts

Dinner: Moroccan-Inspired Apple and Chicken Couscous

Dessert: Sinful Baked Apples with Yogurt Sauce

Day Seven

Breakfast: Pomegranate Berry Smoothie

Midmorning Snack: 1/2 cup sliced strawberries and 1/2 cup nonfat vanilla yogurt

Lunch: Salmon-Infused Waldorf Salad

Midafternoon Snack: Cherry Almond Oat Muffin

Dinner: Whole-Wheat Vegetable Pita Pizza

Dessert: Organic Strawberry Banana Cupcake

Foods That Enhance Your Root Chakra

Fruits and vegetables that contain red pigments and/or skins are excellent ways to support your first energy center and your overall health. In addition, proteins that contain red pigments are beneficial to your root chakra. Some fruits and vegetables with red pigments include the following:

- Apples
- Beets
- Cherries
- Cranberries
- Pink grapefruit
- Pomegranates
- Radicchio
- Radishes
- Raspberries
- Red peppers
- Rhubarb
- Strawberries
- Tomatoes
- Watermelon

Proteins with red pigments include:

- Nuts and seeds
- Salmon
- Tuna

Root Chakra Recipes

Here are this week's gourmet recipes that will enhance your root chakra.

Beet Soup with Carrots and Goat Cheese

Yield: 4 servings   *Prep time:* 10 minutes
Cook time: 2 hours   *Serving size:* 1 cup

4 medium beets

2 cups vegetable stock

4 carrots, chopped

3 sprigs thyme, stems
    removed

5 sprigs sage, fresh

2 sprigs rosemary, fresh

Dash cinnamon

Salt and pepper

½ cup goat cheese,
    softened

2 shallots, chopped

2 garlic cloves, minced

Each serving has:
234 calories
34 g carbohydrates
8 g fat
8 g fiber
10 g protein

1. Boil beets in a large pot of salted water for approximately 2 hours or until tender. Allow beets to cool for 5 minutes.

2. Peel beets and place into a food processor. Add stock, carrots, thyme, sage, rosemary, cinnamon, salt, and pepper. Blend until smooth.

3. Strain mixture through a sieve. In large stockpot over medium-high heat, cook soup mixture for 15 minutes, stirring frequently.

4. In a separate bowl, mix goat cheese with shallots and garlic.

5. Arrange cheese mixture into round shape. Place round cheese shape into a soup bowl and gently ladle soup around it.

6. Garnish with sage or parsley.

Better Than Pizza Salad

Yield: 4 servings   *Prep time:* 5 minutes
Cook time: 13 minutes   *Serving size:* 1 slice

1 store purchased whole-wheat 10-inch pizza crust, prepared

4 oz. olive oil

2 cloves fresh garlic, minced

½ TB. fresh basil

5 cups romaine lettuce leaves

2 medium tomatoes, seeded and diced to ¼-inch pieces

½ cup red onions, seeded and diced

½ cup red and green bell pepper, seeded and diced to ¼-inch pieces

5 mushroom caps, sliced

¼ cup pitted ripe olive, thinly sliced

¼ cup Italian salad dressing, low-calorie

1 cup Mozzarella cheese, shredded

¼ cup Parmesan cheese, grated

Each serving has:
209 calories
16 g carbohydrates
12 g fat
7 g fiber
14 g protein

1. Preheat the oven to 425°F.

2. Combine oil, garlic, and 1/4 tablespoon basil in a bowl. Mix well.

3. Brush garlic mixture over prepared pizza crust, and sprinkle remaining 1/4 tablespoon basil over crust.

4. Place crust on the bottom rack of the oven and bake for 12 to 15 minutes or until crust is golden brown.

5. While crust is baking, place lettuce, tomatoes, onions, peppers, mushrooms, olives, and Italian salad dressing into a large bowl and toss.

6. Remove crust from oven. Immediately sprinkle with half of Mozzarella and Parmesan cheeses. Top with salad and vegetable mixture.

7. Top with remaining Mozzarella and Parmesan cheeses, slice into four equal wedges with a pizza cutter, and serve immediately.

Cheesy Baked Chicken with Chakra Salsa

Yield: 4 to 6 servings   *Prep time:* 10 minutes
Cook time: 30 minutes   *Serving size:* 4 to 6 ounces

1 lb. chicken, boned and
    skinned
1 TB. chili powder
½ cup sliced onion
½ cup sliced red bell pepper
2 oz. fresh cilantro, chopped

4 cups Homemade
    Chakra Salsa (recipe
    in this chapter)
1 cup cheddar cheese,
    shredded

Each serving has:
245 calories
15 g fat
4 g fiber
17 g protein

1. Preheat the oven to 375°F. Grease a shallow baking dish with nonstick vegetable cooking spray.

2. While the oven is preheating, heat the large skillet. Grease a large skillet with nonstick vegetable spray prior to searing the chicken on the stove on medium-high heat.

3. Evenly coat chicken breast with chili powder and sear each side of chicken in the pan.

4. Remove chicken from the skillet and arrange in the baking pan.

5. In the skillet, sauté onions and peppers for 4 to 5 minutes, until slightly browned and tender.

6. Pour onion and pepper mixture and Chakra Salsa over chicken.

7. Bake in the oven for 35 minutes or until chicken reaches an internal temperature of 165°F.

8. Top chicken with shredded cheddar cheese. Bake for additional 10 minutes.

9. Optional: Serve with shredded lettuce, chopped tomatoes, chilled sour cream, or Chakra Guacamole (recipe in Chapter 4).

Cherry Almond Oat Muffins

Yield: 12 servings   *Prep time:* 35 minutes
Cook time: 18 minutes   *Serving size:* 1 muffin

1 cup cultured buttermilk, low-fat

1 cup quick-cooking oats

1 large egg, beaten

½ cup dark brown sugar

1 cup whole-wheat pastry flour

1 tsp. baking powder

½ tsp. baking soda

¼ tsp. ground cinnamon

½ tsp. salt

⅓ cup canola oil

¾ cup dried cherries

½ cup almonds, chopped

Each serving has:
222 calories
30 g carbohydrates
10 g fat
3 g fiber
4 g protein

1. Preheat the oven to 400°F. Grease 12 standard muffin tins with non-stick vegetable cooking spray.

2. Pour buttermilk into a large bowl, and gradually add oats. Stir oat mixture. Allow mixture to sit for 30 minutes.

3. Add well-beaten egg and brown sugar to buttermilk and oats mixture. Stir well.

4. In a separate bowl, whisk whole-wheat pastry flour, baking powder, baking soda, cinnamon, and salt. Stir until well combined. Add above dry ingredients to buttermilk and oat mixture. Stir until moistened. Add oil, dried cherries, and almonds. Stir until well blended.

5. Fill the muffin tins until about ⅔ full. Bake for 18 to 20 minutes or until a toothpick inserted in center of muffin comes out clean.

Cottage Cheese Apple Pancakes

Yield: 8 servings   *Prep time:* 5 minutes
Cook time: 10 minutes   *Serving size:* 2 small pancakes

1 cup whole-wheat pastry flour

1 tsp. cinnamon

1½ tsp. baking powder

1 tsp. orange zest

1 cup milk, skim

1 cup cottage cheese, low-fat

4 egg whites

½ cup apples, diced small

Each serving has:
99 calories
15 g carbohydrates
1 g fat
2 g fiber
8 g protein

1. Place whole-wheat flour, cinnamon, baking powder, and orange zest in a medium-size bowl and stir well. Gradually add milk, cottage cheese, egg whites, and apples. Mix thoroughly.

2. Grease a skillet or griddle with nonstick vegetable cooking spray. Heat skillet on medium-high heat.

3. For each pancake, pour 3 tablespoons batter on the skillet or griddle. Cook on each side for 2 minutes or until pancake is bubbly and edges are golden. Serve immediately.

4. Optional: Serve pancakes topped with fresh, peeled, chopped apples, sliced strawberries, or a dollop of nonfat yogurt.

Homemade Chakra Salsa

Yield: 8 servings   *Prep time:* 15 minutes
Cook time: None; refrigerate overnight.   *Serving size:* 3 ounces

1 (15 oz.) can black-eyed peas

1 (15 oz.) can black beans

1 (15 oz.) can whole-kernel sweet corn, drained (or use fresh)

1 (4 oz.) can green chiles, chopped

1 (15 oz.) can diced tomatoes (or use fresh)

1 cup Italian salad dressing, low-calorie

1 large onion, diced small

¾ cup green pepper, seeded and diced small

½ cup yellow pepper, seeded and diced small

½ cup red pepper, seeded and diced small

¾ cup fresh cilantro, diced fine

Each serving has:
59 calories
8 g carbohydrates
3 g fat
2 g fiber
1 g protein

1. Mix black-eyed peas, black beans, corn, green chiles, diced tomatoes, and Italian salad dressing in a large bowl. Gradually stir in onion, green pepper, yellow pepper, red pepper, and cilantro. Seal and store in an airtight container overnight in the refrigerator before serving.

2. Serve with carrot sticks, celery sticks, and whole-wheat crackers.

Italian Egg-White Frittata

Yield: 1 serving   *Prep time:* 6 minutes
Cook time: 5 minutes   *Serving size:* 1 omelet

4 egg whites

1 TB. green peppers, diced fine

1 TB. red peppers, diced fine

1 TB. green onions

1 TB. black olives, pitted and chopped

2 TB. Mozzarella cheese, part skim milk, shredded

Each serving has:
123 calories
4 g carbohydrates
3 g fat
1 g fiber
18 g protein

1. Combine green and red pepper, green onions, and black olives in a small bowl.

2. Separate egg whites from yolk. Discard yolks. Whisk egg whites.

3. Spray a skillet with nonstick vegetable cooking spray and place on medium-high heat.

4. When the pan is hot, place green and red pepper, onion, and olive mixture in the pan and cook for 1 to 2 minutes.

5. Pour egg whites into the skillet. Cook for approximately 4 minutes, stirring constantly. Sprinkle with cheese. Cook for an additional minute or until cheese is melted. Fold onto a plate and serve immediately.

Mike's Bean Salad with Red Peppers and Feta Cheese

Yield: 6 servings   *Prep time:* 10 minutes   *Marinate time:* 1 hour
Cook time: None   *Serving size:* 1 cup

1 cup canned light red kidney beans, rinsed

1 cup white beans, rinsed

1 cup dark red beans, rinsed

2 medium red bell peppers, diced small

1 oz. fresh cilantro, chopped fine

2 TB. fresh garlic, chopped fine

¼ tsp. cumin powder

1 medium red onion, diced small

½ cup red wine vinegar

¼ cup olive oil

½ cup canned whole-kernel sweet corn, drained

4 whole leaves red leaf lettuce, washed

1 cup feta cheese, crumbled

Salt and white pepper

Each serving has:
431 calories
55 g carbohydrates
15 g fat
16 g fiber
22 g protein

1. Combine beans, red peppers, cilantro, garlic, cumin powder, onion, vinegar, olive oil, and corn in a large bowl, and toss well.

2. Let stand in the refrigerator, covered, for at least 1 hour before serving.

3. Drain excess liquid from salad.

4. Divide salad into 4 portions. Serve on bed of red leaf lettuce. Top each serving with crumbled feta cheese. Salt and pepper to taste.

Moroccan-Inspired Apple and Chicken Couscous

Yield: 6 servings   *Prep time:* 15 minutes
Cook time: 35 minutes   *Serving size:* 1 cup

1 lb. chicken breast halves, skinned and boned

2 large lemons, zested and juiced

1½ cups water

Salt and pepper

1 cup couscous, dry

½ cup fresh peas

2 large carrots, shredded

½ cup golden raisins

½ tsp. cinnamon

½ cup fresh basil, chopped fine

2 large apples, sliced

½ cup almonds, chopped

½ cup cherry tomato, chopped

Each serving has:
368 calories
49 g carbohydrates
12 g fat
6 g fiber
19 g protein

1. Preheat the oven to 350°F.

2. Arrange chicken in a shallow baking dish greased with nonstick vegetable cooking spray. Pour half lemon zest and half lemon juice over chicken.

3. Bake chicken for approximately 30 minutes or until internal temperature reaches 165°F. After chicken cools, shred or slice into 1-inch pieces.

4. Place water, salt and pepper, and remaining lemon juice in a large saucepan. Bring to boil.

5. Add couscous, peas, carrots, raisins, cinnamon, and basil to the boiling saucepan. Cover and simmer for 5 minutes.

6. Remove from heat. Stir well. Allow mixture to stand for 5 minutes.

7. Add sliced apple, shredded chicken, almonds, cherry tomatoes, and remaining lemon zest to mixture. Serve immediately.

Organic Strawberry Banana Cupcakes

Yield: 24 servings   *Prep time:* 10 minutes
Cook time: 13 minutes   *Serving size:* 1 cupcake

6 TB. light butter

2 bananas, ripe and mashed

8 large strawberries, sliced, mashed

1 egg, beaten

⅓ cup milk, skim

2 TB. honey, organic

2 cups whole-wheat pastry flour

¼ tsp. baking soda

1 tsp. cinnamon

½ cup unsweetened organic applesauce

⅓ cup golden raisins

2 bananas, sliced, for decoration

8 large strawberries, sliced, for decoration

Each serving has:
132 calories
24 g carbohydrates
4 g fat
4 g fiber
2 g protein

1. Preheat oven to 400° F.

2. Cream butter, mashed banana, and mashed strawberries in large bowl. Gradually add egg, milk, honey, flour, baking soda, cinnamon, and applesauce to the mixture. When well-blended, gently stir in golden raisins.

3. Evenly divide mixture between 24 cupcake tins lined with paper cupcake holders.

4. Bake for 13-16 minutes or until toothpick inserted into middle of cupcake comes out clean.

5. Remove from oven and cool completely. Decorate with sliced banana and strawberries.

Pomegranate Berry Smoothie

Yield: 2 servings   *Prep time:* 5 minutes
Cook time: None   *Serving size:* 2 cups

1½ cups pomegranate juice

1 cup vanilla yogurt, nonfat

1 cup blueberries

1 TB. honey

1 banana, peeled

1 TB. flaxseed oil

Each serving has:

334 calories

79 g carbohydrates

1 g fat

3 g fiber

8 g protein

1. Place pomegranate juice, yogurt, blueberries, honey, banana, and flaxseed oil in a blender.

2. Purée on high speed until thoroughly blended. Serve immediately.

Root Vegetables Drenched in Honey

Yield: 6 servings   *Prep time:* 5 minutes
Cook time: 60 minutes   *Serving size:* 1½ cups

3 cups sweet potatoes, chopped

2 cups carrots, sliced 1-inch thick

1 cup turnips, chopped

2 cloves garlic, pressed

3 shallots, halved

1 TB. cinnamon

1 TB. kosher salt

Pepper

¾ cup honey, organic

¼ cup extra-virgin olive oil

Each serving has:
307 calories
58 g carbohydrates
9 g fat
4 g fiber
2 g protein

1. Preheat the oven to 425°F.

2. Combine sweet potatoes, carrots, turnips, garlic, and shallots in a shallow baking dish coated with nonstick vegetable oil spray. Sprinkle with cinnamon, salt, and pepper and pour honey and olive oil over vegetables.

3. Roast for 1 hour, stirring once halfway through cooking time.

4. Drizzle with additional honey, if desired.

Salmon-Infused Waldorf Salad

Yield: 4 servings   *Prep time:* 5 minutes
Cook time: None   *Serving size:* 4 ounces

½ cup mayonnaise, imita-
tion, fat-free

14 oz. salmon fillet, cooked
and mashed

⅓ cup walnuts, chopped

1 TB. lemon juice

3 stalks celery, diced fine

½ tsp. thyme

½ tsp. black pepper

1 large apple, diced fine

4 extra large lettuce
leaves

Each serving has:
235 calories
12 g carbohydrates
11 g fat
2 g fiber
23 g protein

1. In a large bowl, mix mayonnaise, salmon, walnuts, lemon juice, celery, thyme, black pepper, and apple.

2. Place lettuce leaves on a plate and fill each leaf with ¼ salmon mixture. Serve.

Sinful Baked Apples with Yogurt Sauce

Yield: 4 servings   *Prep time:* 5 minutes
Cook time: 35 minutes   *Serving size:* 1 apple

4 apples, cored

3 tsp. cinnamon

¼ tsp. nutmeg

¼ cup raisins, seedless

⅓ cup dark brown sugar

¼ cup maple syrup

½ cup low-fat vanilla yogurt

Each serving has:

259 calories

65 g carbohydrates

1 g fat

5 g fiber

2 g protein

1. Preheat the oven to 375°F. Add ¹/₂-inch water to bottom of a baking dish.

2. Core apples and remove top inch of peel. Cut shallow slit into each apple to prevent bursting.

3. Place apples upright in the baking dish.

4. Combine cinnamon, nutmeg, raisins, and dark brown sugar in a small bowl. Mix well. Spoon mixture into cored center of apples.

5. Bake uncovered for 35 to 40 minutes. While apples are baking, combine maple syrup and yogurt in a small bowl.

6. Remove apples from the oven. Apples should be tender when pierced with a toothpick. Drizzle apples with maple yogurt sauce. Serve immediately.

Strawberry Poppy Seed Salad

Yield: 6 servings   *Prep time:* 7 minutes
Cook time: None   *Serving size:* 4 ounces

2 TB. sugar

3 TB. mayonnaise, imitation, no-cholesterol

2 TB. milk, skim

1 TB. poppy seeds

1 TB. cider vinegar

10 oz. romaine lettuce leaves (can use bagged salad mixture)

1½ cups strawberries, sliced

1 (10 oz.) can mandarin oranges, drained

2 TB. almonds, chopped

Each serving has:
111 calories
14 g carbohydrates
6 g fat
3 g fiber
2 g protein

1. Whisk sugar, mayonnaise, skim milk, poppy seeds, and cider vinegar in a small bowl.

2. Place lettuce in a large bowl. Add strawberries, oranges, and almonds. Add ingredients from the small bowl. Toss and serve immediately.

Sweet and Sour Cherry Slaw

Yield: 8 servings   *Prep time:* 8 minutes
Cook time: None   *Serving size:* 4 ounces

¼ cup granulated sugar

½ tsp. dry mustard

½ tsp. celery seed

Dash salt

⅓ cup vegetable oil

¼ cup lime juice

4 TB. honey

16 oz. coleslaw

1 cup shredded carrot, mixture

1 cup dried cherries

½ cup green onion, chopped

2 TB. sunflower seeds

Each serving has:

260 calories

40 g carbohydrates

12 g fat

3 g fiber

2 g protein

1. To make dressing, combine sugar, dry mustard, celery seed, and salt in a small mixing bowl, and mix well. Whisk in vegetable oil, lime juice, and honey until well blended and sugar is dissolved.

2. Combine coleslaw, carrots, cherries, green onions, and sunflower seeds in a large bowl. Pour dressing mixture over coleslaw mixture. Mix thoroughly until well combined. Refrigerate overnight before serving.

Tortilla Pie with Chakra Salsa

Yield: 6 servings   *Prep time:* 8 minutes
Cook time: 18 minutes   *Serving size:* 1 slice

½ lb. cooked chicken, shredded

19 oz. black beans, rinsed and drained

½ cup nonfat sour cream

16 oz. Homemade Chakra Salsa (recipe in this chapter)

¼ cup fresh cilantro, chopped fine

5 (10-inch) whole-wheat flour tortillas, low-fat

2 cups Monterey Jack cheese, reduced-fat, shredded

Each serving has:
508 calories
49 g carbohydrates
18 g fat
8 g fiber
33 g protein

1. Preheat the oven to 425°F.

2. In a large bowl, combine chicken, black beans, sour cream, salsa, and cilantro.

3. Grease bottom of a shallow baking pan with nonstick vegetable cooking spray. Place 1 tortilla in the greased pan. Top tortilla with 1½ cups chicken and bean mixture and ½ cup cheese.

4. Layer three more times. Place tortilla on top.

5. Bake in the oven for 18 to 20 minutes, or until filling is hot and cheese melts.

Whole-Wheat Vegetable Pita Pizzas

Yield: 4 servings   *Prep time:* 5 minutes
Cook time: 10 minutes   *Serving size:* 1 slice

4 (7-inch) whole-wheat pita bread rounds

1 TB. olive oil

1 lb. fresh tomatoes, cored and sliced

2 TB. fresh basil, chopped

3 tsp. Parmesan cheese, grated

2 cups Mozzarella cheese, part skim milk

2 cups (about 1 large) zucchini, shredded

1 cup green bell pepper, seeded and diced small

4 mushrooms, sliced

4 black olives, pitted and sliced

¼ cup sweet red onion, diced small

1½ tsp. Italian seasoning

Each serving has:
239 calories
12 g carbohydrates
14 g fat
2 g fiber
18 g protein

1. Preheat the oven to 425°F.

2. Place 4 pita rounds evenly on 2 separate baking sheets.

3. Brush pitas with olive oil. Arrange tomato slices on each pita round, dividing evenly. Sprinkle with basil and Parmesan cheese. Bake for 10 minutes. Remove from the oven.

4. Sprinkle pitas with Mozzarella cheese. Top with zucchini, green pepper, mushrooms, olives, and onion. Bake an additional 10 minutes or until cheese is melted and vegetables are crispy and tender. Serve immediately.

5. Optional: Serve with crushed red pepper and additional Parmesan cheese.

Exercises to Balance Your First Chakra

Here are several personal-growth exercises that will help you attain inner peace during your weight-loss journey.

Breathing Exercises

Breath is something most of us take for granted. It is an involuntary response we rarely think about. Air is one of our basic survival needs. Food and water comprise a mere 10 percent of the human body's daily requirements. An alarming 90 percent of our body's daily requirement is oxygen. Perhaps many people overeat in an effort to nourish an oxygen-starved body! Without breath, human beings can survive approximately 10 minutes.

Most of us do not breathe properly, and deprive ourselves of the vital energy we need to prosper. By training our lungs to effectively take in and dispel air, we can literally transform our lives and our entire chakra system.

The first step to inner peace through breathing is simply to notice your own breathing patterns. Sit quietly in a space where you will not be disturbed. Become aware of your body drawing in air. Do not attempt to change or alter anything. Simply notice your own unique and conditioned way of inhaling. Gently observe how you exhale. Do you empty your lungs completely, or do you hold your breath? Take 10 minutes to notice your breath.

Our breath is often an accurate reflection of how we live our lives. For example, does your rapid, uneven breathing mirror your chaotic and fast-paced lifestyle? In your journal, write any thoughts, feelings, and behaviors that this exercise stirred in you. Keeping a journal is an excellent way to lose weight and feel peaceful. Journal writing simply involves writing your thoughts, feelings, and experiences down on paper. It is a beneficial tool to connect with yourself and get in touch with your innermost desires and emotions.

Yoga teacher Dawn Mehan teaches that there are five qualities to good breath. Life-sustaining breath is deep, smooth, even, without sound, and without pause. Does your breath embody these qualities? The following exercises are designed to help you attain healthy breathing patterns that will ground and support your root chakra center. These breathing exercises are based on techniques taught by Dawn Mehan.

Breathing from Your Belly

With your eyes closed, place your right hand over your heart center, and place your left hand over your belly. Placing your hand over your heart is an act of self-love that provides an instant sense of tranquility. By placing your hand over your belly, you will be able to sense your deep breaths and learn how to breathe more effectively.

Allow yourself to breathe normally for three complete breaths. When you are ready, gently inhale, filling your belly with a long, cleansing breath and sensing this breath with your left hand. Now, fill your belly with air, then fill your lower lungs with air, and finally fill your upper lungs with air. Imagine that you are filling a glass with clean, refreshing water. Pour the water from the bottom of your belly to the top of your lungs. As you exhale, imagine that you are emptying the same glass of water. First, empty the air from your upper lungs, then from your lower lungs, and, finally, empty your belly. Practice this for 10 minutes.

Relaxing Breath

Sit in a comfortable position. Make sure that you are seated in a posture that you do not have to struggle to maintain.

Close your eyes. Allow yourself to sink into your chair or the floor. Relax your body and clear your mind of any thoughts or worries. As you close your eyes, feel how totally and completely supported you are in this moment. Slowly inhale as you count to three. Without pausing between breaths, immediately exhale as you silently count to five.

This simple exercise guarantees relaxation. As you inhale, you are stimulating your sympathetic nervous system. Your sympathetic nervous system mediates your body's natural responses to stress and physical activity by increasing your heart rate, your blood pressure, and your muscle tone.

As you exhale, you are engaging your parasympathetic nervous system. Responsible for rest, sleep, and digestion, the parasympathetic nervous system decreases your heart rate, blood pressure, and muscle tone. This simple breathing exercise lowers your heart rate, blood pressure, and muscle tone by drawing on the wisdom of your own body.

Healing Breath

Lie down on the floor or in your bed. With your eyes closed, practice breathing naturally for a few moments.

Either silently or aloud, ask yourself what part of your body most needs healing in this moment. Place your dominant hand over the area of your body that requests therapeutic touch. This area may be injured, infected, or simply just calls out for your mindfulness.

Place your other hand on your abdomen. Slowly inhale.

As you inhale, visualize a healing energy flowing into your dominant hand. Picture this energy as a repairing and rejuvenating white light. With each inhalation, imagine this healing light purifying and cleansing this area of your body. As you exhale, imagine the pain and negativity washing out of your body and your life. Continue breathing deeply and visualizing the healing white light for 10 minutes.

One Hundred Ways You Are Supported in This Moment

If you frequently find yourself fretting over your bank balance or worrying about your children's well-being, this exercise will be particularly useful for rooting your first chakra. This activity can be done while you are meditating, or you may choose to record this exercise in your journal. A surefire way to reconnect with a strong sense of security and balance your first chakra is to remind yourself that you are completely supported by the universe. Dr. Valerie Hunt, a metaphysical healer, teaches that visualizing your chakras spinning can help bring them back into alignment. The following exercise will strengthen your first energy center and help eliminate a sense of struggle from your life.

Find a quiet place where you can do this exercise without being interrupted. Prior to beginning, take a few deep, cleansing breaths. Gently close your eyes. Spend a few minutes visualizing a red ball spinning clockwise in your pelvic area. If you have troubling seeing the color red, imagine a large red apple in the center of your pelvic floor. Focus on breathing in and breathing out, as you continue to visualize this large red ball spinning clockwise in your groin area. Continue breathing and seeing the color red for 10 minutes.

List 100 ways you are supported by the universe in this moment. You may list "your 100 ways" aloud, silently in your mind, or in your journal.

Think about all of your needs that have been met today without any effort or struggling on your part. Remember all of the wonderful gifts you have been given today that did not cost you a thing. Be creative with your list. Attempt to list 100 items effortlessly.

If you are having difficulty thinking of things to add to your list, do not worry or think negatively. You may repeat items until you think of new ways that the universe supports you. Release any thoughts of self-judgment and perfectionism.

Here is a sample list to help you get started.

- Today I am provided with a free, limitless supply of oxygen that nourishes my lungs.

- My body releases carbon dioxide and other toxins without my having to willfully discharge them.

- My heart pumps my blood effectively and nourishes my whole body, without my thinking about it.

After you complete your own list, take a few deep, cleansing breaths. The next time you find yourself feeling anxious, repeat this exercise to remedy your feelings of insecurity.

Get Physical! Stimulate Your Root Chakra

Exercise is a necessary component to a healthy lifestyle. You probably were aware of that before you picked up this book. But did you know that specific exercises might not only help you shed pounds but also help you gain happiness and prosperity?

Get Grounded

Brisk walking is an excellent way to ground your root chakra and bring your first energy center into alignment. Walking is also a wonderful exercise for beginners and serves as a foundation for the other exercises in this book. I recommend taking at least three 45-minute walks this week, preferably outdoors. As you walk, feel the soles of your feet connect with the earth. Visualize a silver rope that extends from your pelvis, always anchoring you to the earth and supporting you.

Stomping and jumping rope are also great effective chakra stimulators. Phylamena lila Desy, an intuitive counselor encourages her clients to put on some loud, revitalizing music and stomp vigorously on the floor for at least

20 minutes. You may alternate stomping and jumping as you see fit. Many people feel as if they are releasing pent up rage during this exercise. Allow yourself to experience any feelings that arise, without fear or judgment.

I also recommend doing squats to get the energy flowing to your root chakra. Keep your back straight, and bend your knees as you gently lower your body to the ground. Pay attention to your breathing as you squat. Make sure that you are not holding your breath. Make a conscious effort to breath in and out through your nose.

Yoga

Yoga is an ancient art and science that has existed for over 2000 years. Its major purpose is to bring your chakra system into balance and help you discover your true self.

Yoga teacher Dawn Mehan affirms that the Mountain pose, known as Tadasana in Sanskrit, is an effective way to stimulate your first chakra center. To assume the Mountain pose, first stand with your feet parallel and your shoulders rolled back and down. Make sure that your weight is evenly distributed throughout your entire body. Rock back and forth on your heels for a few moments and gradually come to a standstill.

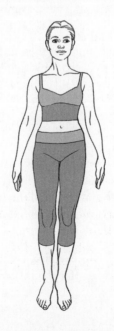

Mountain Pose

Lift your sternum toward the ceiling, and allow your arms to gently hang by your sides. Keep your belly soft and remember to keep breathing. Try to hold the pose for three minutes as you focus only on your breathing. The Mountain pose renews your sense of equilibrium and balance. This yoga pose can be done virtually anywhere.

Try getting in this posture the next time you find yourself in line at the grocery or post office. Notice how alive and grounded your whole body feels after you do this pose. Pay specific attention to the energy in your pelvic region.

Root Chakra Body Scanning and Muscle Relaxation Technique

Lie down on the floor or in your bed. Gently close your eyes and clear your mind of any thoughts and worries. Take a few deep, cleansing breaths. Welcome everything you are experiencing right now.

Focus all of your attention on your feet. Gently squeeze and tighten all the muscles in your feet for seven seconds. Continue to hold the tension. Now, all at once, relax and let go. Breathe as if you are breathing from your feet. Become aware of every sensation that exists in your feet. What message do your feet have for you? Spend as much time as you need to simply focus on your feet.

Next, gradually shift your attention to your lower calves. How do your calves feel? Are you are able to rock them back and forth without pain or discomfort? Do they feel loose and relaxed? Now stiffen your calve muscles and hold the tension for seven seconds. All at once, let go and relax your calves. If your calves could talk, what would they say now? Fill your calves with a healing breath.

Continue this exercise as you slowly work you way up your entire body. Be sure to isolate the tension in each muscle group for at least seven seconds. Be gentle with yourself and decrease the tension if you feel pain. Take time listening to your body and scanning it for any messages that you need to hear.

After you have completed this exercise, breathe deeply for a few minutes. At the end of this exercise, offer thanks to your body for the support it gives to you.

2

Your Sacral Chakra

The second chakra is known as the sacral chakra. It is represented by the color orange. Physically this chakra is located in the uterus in women and near the spleen in men. Known as the seat of creation, the second chakra is closely related to sexuality and conception. The second chakra also helps us to identify and process our emotions and feelings. This energy center is enhanced by wearing orange clothing and gemstones.

A dysfunctional second chakra can cause weight gain related to emotional eating. Many people eat as a substitute for sexual or emotional satisfaction. Once someone secures his survival needs by grounding the first chakra, he will seek pleasure through the second chakra.

People with an unbalanced second chakra may fear intimacy, have problems with impotency or infertility, or resist change. In addition, many people with a blocked second chakra have an inability to feel pleasure or create the life they truly want. Guilt and sexual repression can become lifelong problems for a person who never resolves her sacral chakra issues.

After completing this week's exercises and eating plan, you will feel more like the creative, sensual, and emotionally healthy individual that you were destined to be. The goal of this chapter is to help you get in touch with your emotions and eating habits and your ability to create pleasure in your life. Water is the element most closely associated with the second chakra.

This week, focus on increasing your water intake to at least 10 8-ounce glasses per day, as you continue to incorporate more fresh fruits and vegetables into your diet.

Let's get started by taking a look at this week's eating plan.

SACRAL CHAKRA SEVEN-DAY EATING PLAN

Day One

Breakfast: Mango Peach Smoothie
Midmorning Snack: 1 large orange
Lunch: Papaya Passion Salad
Midafternoon Snack: $1/4$ cup pumpkin seeds
Dinner: Tilapia Scampi
Dessert: Healthy Carrot Cake

Day Two

Breakfast: Peach Kiwi Salad
Midmorning Snack: 10 carrot sticks
Lunch: Sacral Delight Hummus and Whole-Wheat Pita Squares
Midafternoon Snack: 1 small tangerine
Dinner: Apricot Almond Chicken
Dessert: All Natural Pumpkin Fudge

Day Three

Breakfast: Pumpkin Orange Bread
Midmorning Snack: $1/2$ cup nonfat cottage cheese and $1/2$ cup dried apricots
Lunch: Sweet Potato Soup
Midafternoon Snack: 1 peach
Dinner: Pumpkin Pasta Primavera
Dessert: Peach Sorbet

Day Four

Breakfast: Mango Peach Smoothie
Midmorning Snack: $1/4$ cup almonds
Lunch: Mandarin and Hazelnut Spinach Salad
Midafternoon Snack: 1 peach

Dinner: Tilapia Scampi

Dessert: Carrot and Orange Salad

Day Five

Breakfast: Peach Kiwi Salad

Midmorning Snack: 1 slice cantaloupe with $1/2$ TB. honey

Lunch: Sacral Delight Hummus

Midafternoon Snack: 1 large apple

Dinner: Sweet Potato Soup

Dessert: All Natural Pumpkin Fudge

Day Six

Breakfast: Pumpkin Orange Bread

Midmorning Snack: $1/2$ cup nonfat yogurt and 1 peach

Lunch: Maple Glazed Butternut Squash

Midafternoon Snack: 1 mango

Dinner: Apricot Almond Chicken

Dessert: Healthy Carrot Cake

Day Seven

Breakfast: Mango Peach Smoothie

Midmorning Snack: 1 slice cantaloupe

Lunch: Papaya Passion Salad

Midafternoon Snack: $1/2$ cup Sacral Delight Hummus and carrot sticks

Dinner: Mandarin and Hazelnut Spinach Salad

Dessert: Peach Sorbet

Foods That Enhance Your Sacral Chakra

Fruits and vegetables that contain orange pigments and/or skins are excellent ways to support your second energy center and your overall health.

Some fruits and vegetables with orange-colored skins and pigments include the following:

- Apricots
- Cantaloupe
- Carrots
- Mangos
- Papaya
- Peaches
- Persimmons
- Pumpkins
- Squash
- Sweet potatoes
- Tangerines

Sacral Chakra Recipes

Here are this week's gourmet recipes to enhance your second chakra and accelerate weight loss.

Mango Peach Smoothie

Yield: 1 serving   *Prep time:* 5 minutes
Cook time: None   *Serving size:* 1 cup

1 large mango, peeled and chopped

1 large peach, peeled and chopped

1 TB. organic honey

1 TB. flaxseed oil

1 cup vanilla yogurt, nonfat

½ cup skim milk

½ cup ice cubes

Each serving has:
245 calories
55 g carbohydrates
1 g fat
3 g fiber
9 g protein

1. Place mango, peach, honey, flaxseed oil, yogurt, milk, and ice cubes in a blender.

2. Purée on high speed until blended thoroughly. Serve immediately.

Sweet Potato Soup

Yield: 8 servings   *Prep time:* 10 minutes
Cook time: 30 minutes   *Serving size:* 1 cup

4 cups vegetable stock,
   organic, ready-to-serve

3 large sweet potatoes,
   peeled and chopped

2 celery ribs, chopped

1 large Vidalia or Spanish
   onion, chopped fine

1 tsp. cinnamon

2 tsp. fresh tarragon

½ tsp. nutmeg

1 bay leaf

2 cups skim milk

Salt and pepper

½ cup sour cream,
   fat-free

Each serving has:
121 calories
19 g carbohydrates
4 g fat
2 g fiber
4 g protein

1. Combine vegetable stock, sweet potatoes, celery, onions, cinnamon, tarragon, nutmeg, and bay leaf in a large pot over high heat and bring to a boil.

2. Reduce heat and simmer until vegetables are tender, 25 to 30 minutes.

3. Discard bay leaf. Purée soup in a food processor or a blender. Return to the pot on the stove.

4. Add milk, and bring to a simmer. Ladle into portions.

5. Garnish each portion with dollop of fat-free sour cream. Salt and pepper to taste.

Papaya Passion Salad

Yield: 8 servings   *Prep time:* 20 minutes
Cook time: None   *Serving size:* 1 cup

½ cup extra-virgin olive oil

¼ cup lemon juice, fresh-squeezed

1 medium onion, minced

1 large papaya, chopped and pitted

1 large peach, chopped and pitted

1 head romaine lettuce, washed, dried, and chopped

1 pint strawberries, sliced

⅓ cup almonds, halved

Each serving has:
208 calories
13 g carbohydrates
16 g fat
4 g fiber
4 g protein

1. Combine oil, lemon juice, minced onion, papaya, and peach in a large bowl. Toss well. Let stand for 10 to 15 minutes.

2. Drain excess liquid from papaya mixture.

3. Combine lettuce with papaya mixture. Toss well.

4. Place 1-cup portions onto plates. Top with strawberries and almonds. Serve.

Tilapia Scampi

Yield: 6 servings   *Prep time:* 10 minutes
Cook time: 10 minutes   *Serving size:* 5 ounces

1½ lb. tilapia fillets

1 cup whole-wheat flour

3 TB. olive oil

3 large cloves garlic, minced

¼ cup dry white wine

2 tsp. lemon juice

2 tsp. minced parsley

¼ tsp. oregano

Salt and pepper

3 fresh basil leaves, chopped

3 cups cooked brown rice

Each serving has:
599 calories
89 g carbohydrates
10 g fat
2 g fiber
32 g protein

1. Rinse each tilapia fillet in cold water. Pat dry lightly. Dredge in flour. Shake fillet to remove excess flour, and set aside.

2. In a large skillet, heat olive oil over medium-high heat. Add garlic to the skillet and cook until lightly browned.

3. Add tilapia fillets to skillet. Cook on both sides, making sure to lightly brown each side.

4. Add wine, lemon juice, parsley, oregano, salt, and pepper. Simmer until heated through. Garnish with basil.

5. Serve over brown rice.

Carrot and Orange Salad

Yield: 2 servings   *Prep time:* 10 minutes
Cook time: None; refrigerate overnight.   *Serving size:* 12 ounces

2 large carrots, shredded

1 (15 oz.) can mandarin oranges, rinsed and drained

½ cup golden seedless raisins

1 TB. honey

2 TB. orange juice, freshly squeezed

½ tsp. ground cinnamon

Each serving has:
241 calories
62 g carbohydrates
1 g fat
7 g fiber
3 g protein

1. Place shredded carrots, oranges, raisins, honey, orange juice, and cinnamon in a large bowl. Toss well.

2. Place the bowl in refrigerator overnight to allow flavors to blend together. Serve.

Pumpkin Orange Bread

Yield: 12 servings   *Prep time:* 10 minutes
Cook time: 45 minutes   *Serving size:* 1 slice

1 cup pumpkin, mashed,
cooked or canned

1 cup sugar

½ cup brown sugar

1 whole egg

1 egg white

½ cup orange juice

1 teaspoon vanilla extract

¼ cup flaxseed oil

1¾ cups whole-wheat
pastry flour

2 tsp. baking powder

½ tsp. ground cloves

½ TB. nutmeg

½ tsp. cinnamon

½ cup dried cranberries,
chopped

Each serving has:
170 calories
38 carbohydrates
3 g fat
3 g fiber
3 g protein

1. Preheat oven to 350°F. Stir mashed pumpkin, sugar, brown sugar, eggs, orange juice, vanilla extract, and flaxseed oil. Slowly add whole-wheat flour, baking powder, cloves, nutmeg, and cinnamon to mixture. Stir until well blended. Fold in dried cranberries.

2. Grease 9×5 bread pan with nonstick vegetable oil cooking spray. Pour batter evenly into pan.

3. Bake 45 minutes. Remove from oven when toothpick inserted into center of bread comes out clean. Cool in pan for 10 minutes and transfer to wire rack.

Peach Kiwi Salad

Yield: 6 servings   *Prep time:* 15 minutes
Cook time: None   *Serving size:* 12 ounces

1 large peach, pitted and peeled, cut into ½-inch pieces

1 large mango, peeled and cut into ½-inch pieces

1 large pineapple, peeled, cored, and sliced into ½-inch pieces

2 kiwifruits, peeled and sliced into ¼-inch pieces

1 TB. fresh lime juice

2 TB. lime zest

1 tsp. fresh garlic, grated

1 tsp. red chili peppers, chopped fine, seeded and chopped

1 TB. fresh basil, chopped

Each serving has:
86 calories
22 g carbohydrates
1 g fat
3 g fiber
1 g protein

1. Place peaches, mangos, pineapple, and kiwi in a large bowl. Gently toss.

2. Add lime juice, lime zest, fresh garlic, and chili peppers. Toss until fruit is well coated. Garnish with basil.

3. Serve immediately, or refrigerate until ready to serve.

Mandarin and Hazelnut Spinach Salad

Yield: 4 servings   *Prep time:* 15 minutes
Cook time: None   *Serving size:* 2 cups

8 cups spinach leaves

1 cup fresh mushrooms, sliced

22 oz. mandarin orange sections, drained and rinsed

¼ cup feta cheese, crumbled

¼ cup extra-virgin olive oil

¼ cup Balsamic vinegar

2 TB. hazelnuts, chopped

Each serving has:
270 calories
24 g carbohydrates
19 g fat
6 g fiber
6 g protein

1. Place spinach, mushrooms, mandarin oranges, and feta cheese in a large bowl. Gently toss.

2. Drizzle salad with vinegar and oil.

3. Top salad with hazelnuts, and serve.

Maple Glazed Butternut Squash

Yield: 4 servings   *Prep time:* 15 minutes
Cook time: 50 minutes   *Serving size:* ¼ pound

½ cup maple syrup
¼ tsp. cinnamon
⅛ tsp. ground cardamom
2 TB. packed brown sugar
Salt and pepper

1 lb. butternut squash, diced medium
2 TB. lemon juice
2 TB. extra-virgin olive oil

Each serving has:
267 calories
43 g carbohydrates
12 g fat
2 g fiber
1 g protein

1. Preheat the oven to 350°F.

2. In a large mixing bowl, combine maple syrup, cinnamon, cardamom, brown sugar, salt, and pepper.

3. Place squash in the bowl containing mixture. Toss until coated evenly. Place evenly in a baking pan.

4. Drizzle lemon juice and olive oil over top of squash.

5. Bake, uncovered, for 45 minutes or until tender.

Pumpkin Pasta Primavera

Yield: 4 servings   *Prep time:* 15 minutes
Cook time: 20 minutes   *Serving size:* 2 cups

1 TB. extra-virgin olive oil

1 large onion, peeled and chopped small

1 large red bell pepper, seeded and chopped small

1 large green bell pepper, seeded and chopped small

3 cloves garlic, peeled and crushed

1 (15 oz.) can pumpkin

8 oz. vegetable stock

2 TB. parsley, chopped fine

4 oz. skim milk

½ tsp. ground nutmeg

Pinch cinnamon

Pinch salt

Pinch black pepper

4 cups hot, cooked whole-wheat pasta

Each serving has:
505 calories
101 g carbohydrates
6 g fat
12 g fiber
20 g protein

1. Heat a skillet over medium-high heat.

2. Sauté oil, onions, red and green peppers, and garlic for 4 to 5 minutes or until vegetables are tender.

3. Add pumpkin and vegetable stock to the pan and bring to boil.

4. Cover and simmer over medium heat for 15 minutes, stirring occasionally.

5. Beat pumpkin with a wooden spoon until it breaks up. Stir in parsley, milk, nutmeg, cinnamon, salt, and pepper.

6. Pour pumpkin sauce over hot whole-wheat pasta, and serve immediately.

Sacral Delight Hummus

Yield: 12 servings   *Prep time:* 10 minutes
Cook time: None   *Serving size:* 2 ounces

2 (15 oz.) cans garbanzo
beans

½ cup tahini

2 TB. nonfat yogurt

6 TB. lemon juice, fresh-
squeezed

3 cloves garlic, pressed

1 tsp. ground cumin

Salt and pepper

Each serving has:
147 calories
19 g carbohydrates
6 g fat
4 g fiber
5 g protein

1. Drain garbanzo beans and reserve liquid.

2. Place beans, tahini, yogurt, lemon juice, garlic, and ground cumin into a food processor.

3. Add ¼ cup reserved liquid from canned beans.

4. Process until mixture is smooth.

5. Serve with carrot sticks, celery sticks, and whole-wheat pita crackers. Salt and pepper to taste.

Apricot Almond Chicken

Yield: 6 servings   *Prep time:* 10 minutes
Cook time: 25 minutes   *Serving size:* 5 ounces

2 TB. extra-virgin olive oil

3 medium Vidalia onions, sliced

1 tsp. chili pepper, minced

1½ tsp. fresh ginger, minced

1½ tsp. fresh garlic, minced

1 tsp. allspice

2 tsp. cinnamon

1 tsp. turmeric

1½ lb. chicken, boned and skinned

1½ cups diced tomatoes

1 cup dried apricot

1 tsp. salt

¾ cup almonds, chopped

Each serving has:
432 calories
24 g carbohydrates
20 g fat
6 g fiber
20 g protein

1. Place olive oil in a large skillet and heat over medium-high heat. Add onions, chili peppers, ginger, garlic, allspice, cinnamon, and turmeric. Sauté for about 6 minutes or until onions are lightly browned and tender.

2. Add chicken to the skillet. Brown chicken on all sides. Gradually stir in tomatoes, apricots, and salt. Cover and simmer on low heat for 15 minutes or until chicken reaches internal temperature of 165°F.

3. Sprinkle with almonds prior to serving.

All Natural Pumpkin Fudge

Yield: 15 servings   *Prep time:* 10 minutes
Cook time: 20 minutes   *Serving size:* 1 small square

1 cup skim milk	Dash salt	*Each serving has:*
2 cups sugar	1 tsp. vanilla	155 calories
2 TB. light corn syrup	½ tsp. cloves	32 g carbohydrates
1 TB. organic honey	4 TB. non-transfat marga-	3 g fat
½ cup pumpkin, cooked and	rine or light butter	Trace fiber
mashed	½ tsp. cinnamon	1 g protein

1. Combine skim milk, sugar, corn syrup, honey, pumpkin, and salt in a large, heavy stock pot. Bring the pot to boil over medium-high heat. When mixture comes to rolling boil, continue stirring for 2 to 5 minutes.

2. Reduce heat. Simmer until mixture reads 236°F on a candy thermometer.

3. Remove from heat. Stir in vanilla, cloves, margarine, and cinnamon. Allow mixture to cool for 20 minutes. Beat mixture until thick, and it loses its glossy finish. Pour mixture in a square dish coated with non-stick vegetable spray. Allow fudge to cool for 2 hours before cutting into pieces.

Healthy Carrot Cake

Yield: 15 servings   *Prep time:* 10 minutes
Cook time: 40 minutes   *Serving size:* 1 slice

2 cups whole-wheat pastry flour

3 tsp. ground cinnamon

2 tsp. baking soda

½ tsp. nutmeg, ground

½ tsp. cloves, ground

6 egg whites, room temperature

1 cup sugar

1 cup unsweetened applesauce

2 TB. organic honey

½ cup cultured buttermilk, low-fat

1½ tsp. vanilla

2 cups shredded carrots

8 oz. canned crushed pineapple, undrained

½ cup raisins

½ cup walnuts, chopped

¼ cup dates, chopped

Each serving has:
203 calories
41 g carbohydrates
3 g fat
4 g fiber
5 g protein

1. Preheat the oven to 350°F. Grease and flour a 13×9-inch baking pan.

2. In a large bowl, mix flour, cinnamon, baking soda, nutmeg, and cloves.

3. In a separate large bowl, beat egg whites until fluffy peak forms. Gradually beat in sugar. Next, slowly beat in applesauce, honey, low-fat buttermilk, and vanilla.

4. Use a wooden spoon to stir flour mixture into egg and applesauce mixture. Next, add carrots, crushed pineapple, raisins, walnuts, and dates.

5. Spread mixture into the greased and floured pan. Bake for 40 minutes or until a toothpick inserted near center of cake comes out clean.

Peach Sorbet

Yield: 4 servings   *Prep time:* 10 minutes
Cook time: None; freeze overnight   *Serving size:* 1 cup

1½ lb. peaches
½ cup granulated sugar

3 TB. lemon juice, fresh-squeezed

Each serving has:
154 calories
32 g carbohydrates
0 fat
3 g fiber
1 g protein

1. Wash peaches, then peel and chop coarse after removing pits.

2. Put peaches and sugar into a food processor. Blend until liquefied.

3. Add lemon juice. Blend for a few seconds longer.

4. Transfer mixture to a metal container and freeze overnight. For best results, place empty metal container in freezer for three hours prior to adding peach sorbet.

5. Scoop out and serve with a topping of fat-free whipped topping and garnish with sprig of fresh mint or cilantro.

Rich and Creamy Carrot Soup

Yield: 3 servings   *Prep time:* 10 minutes
Cook time: 20 minutes   *Serving size:* 1 cup

2 TB. extra-virgin olive oil

1 cup Vidalia onion, chopped fine

1 lb. carrots, sliced, and cooked

2 cups vegetable stock

¼ tsp. ground nutmeg

½ tsp. cinnamon

½ cup orange juice, fresh-squeezed

Salt and pepper, to taste

3 TB. nonfat yogurt

Each serving has:
293 calories
41 g carbohydrates
12 fat
7 g fiber
7 g protein

1. Heat olive oil in a large pan over medium-high heat. Sauté onions until lightly browned and tender.

2. Transfer onions to a large saucepan and add cooked carrots, vegetable stock, nutmeg, and cinnamon.

3. Add orange juice. Heat mixture over medium-high heat for 10 minutes.

4. Transfer mixture to a food processor. Blend until very smooth. Add salt and pepper to taste.

5. Return mixture to the saucepan and bring soup to boil.

6. Garnish with yogurt and serve.

Exercises to Balance Your Sacral Chakra

Let's look at this week's personal-growth exercises that will balance your second energy center.

Journal to Your Dream Life

This week, take the first step toward your ideal body and dream lifestyle. Your second chakra directly reflects your ability to create the life you want for yourself. When you struggle with weight issues, your ability to give birth to the life you desire is very limited. This exercise is a transformative experience, providing you with instant gratification. This helps you quickly identify the areas of your life that are in harmony, and those that are not working.

What Do You Want?

Write down the seven things that you most want to happen in your life. Be creative, and think big. Don't worry about how you will achieve or attain these things. Act as if you can be, do, or have anything you want. Allow yourself to write down those expansive dreams you have not yet given yourself permission to experience. Imagine that anything is possible. Rekindle old dreams and desires from your childhood and adolescence.

If you are having difficulty identifying things you want most in life, make a list of seven things you do not want to experience or have. Spend some more time transforming each item on your "don't want list" into a desired item that gets you excited.

Next, look carefully at your "do want" list. Why do you want to have these experiences, items, or people in your life? How would you feel if you woke up tomorrow to discover that all seven items on your "want list" were granted? At the very core of our beings, most of us simply want to experience happiness and serenity. We believe that if we attain material goods and objects, they will bring us the happiness that eludes us in our everyday lives.

Imagine that in this moment you have everything that you most desire. Feel the happiness. Keep this feeling alive inside of your body. Spend 10 minutes focusing on these joyous feelings. This week, vow to take one small step toward your dream life. For example, if the top item on your list is "Buy an airplane and fly to all seven continents," spend some of your free time researching flying lessons on the Internet. Be adventurous and take a giant leap into your dream life.

Revisit Your Childhood Pleasures

Inside each and every one of us is a small child with a creative heart and soul. Most small children have thriving sacral chakras and enjoy living in the moment. They spend their days involved in creative and imaginative play. As a result of this spontaneous way of being, children experience joyous emotions. This week, spend some time observing a toddler at play. Notice how the small child unabashedly displays her emotions and follows her inner voice. Record your observations and your experience in your journal.

As we mature, we learn from those around us that our desires are not always socially acceptable. From an early age, we are urged to conform to societal norms. Others insist that we share our toys when we want to play alone, urge us to be nice when we feel angry, or demand that we use the toilet before we are truly ready. Misguided parents use food to reward our behavior when we adhere to their standards. This causes confusion, because we begin to view food as a prize instead of as life-sustaining nutrition. As a result, we learn to mask our genuine emotions, and our creativity is diminished.

During adolescence, the voice of our inner self is further silenced, as we are encouraged to constantly look toward the future instead of living in the present. Well-intentioned parents and teachers may steer us away from a profession in the creative arts, and encourage us to pursue a career that will provide us with a stable income and job security. As a result of this conditioning, many adults find themselves unhappy in their personal and professional lives, and they turn to food for comfort.

In your journal, make a list of all of the activities you delighted in when you were a youngster. Think of the things you used to do that made you lose track of time. Don't dismiss items because they seem silly or unproductive.

Examples of pleasurable childhood activities might include roller-skating, finger-painting, playing with toys, dancing to loud music, horseback riding, and playing in a sandbox. After you complete your list, review each item and try to recall the feeling each activity evoked within you. For example, playing with Play-Doh caused you to feel excited as you experienced the endless possibilities of your own creativity.

Spend at least 30 minutes doing the activity that brought you the most pleasure in your childhood. Give yourself permission to be silly and spontaneous. Leave the office a half-hour early to go for an impromptu bike ride or trip to the playground.

Indulge in your favorite childhood activity this week. Notice how your serenity increases and your sense of possibility expands.

Your Pain Spot Versus Your Pleasure Spot

It is human nature to seek pleasure and avoid pain. Your sacral chakra is your gateway to pleasure in the physical world. Its primary function is to help you seek enjoyment and avoid discomfort. Every human behavior has an ultimate payoff or reward. Many destructive behaviors, such as overeating, are misguided attempts to avoid pain in life. Believe it or not, these destructive behaviors offer us a certain type of reward; they protect us in some way. Before advancing further in your journey to permanent weight loss, it is vital for you to understand what you have gained from being overweight, other than just pounds.

For some people, extra pounds serve as a literal shield that protects them from unwanted sexual advances or emotional intimacy. After experiencing childhood sexual abuse, it is common for abuse survivors to gain large amounts of weight in an effort to downplay their physical attractiveness. For most people, this behavior is unconscious and they are not aware of their motives.

Others may gain weight following a major life event such as marriage or childbirth. They have difficulty embracing change, and enjoy comforting themselves by gorging on previously forbidden foods. Yet other people reward themselves for self–sacrifice with food. Self-described food martyrs, they forfeit their heart's desires to care for small children or sick family members. At the end of the day, they reward their self-deprivation by polluting their bodies with the junk food and extra calories they crave. Others use food as a drug, in an attempt to mask unwanted thoughts and feelings.

Maybe you recognize yourself in one of these scenarios. Every one of us has a unique situation and story to tell about our pleasure and our pain. This week, begin your journey to permanent weight loss by journaling about the rewards you have received by being overweight or by overeating.

Next, write about the pain that being overweight has caused you. It is natural to feel angry or outraged while doing this exercise. It can be difficult to acknowledge that the source of your pain also could bring you pleasure. In order for you to make permanent changes, realize that the pain of being overweight needs to outweigh the pleasures of overeating unhealthy foods. Most importantly, being healthy needs to take priority over the deeper payoff, such as masking feelings and avoiding intimacy.

Eat with Your Fingers

Your sacral chakra is stimulated by sensual activities, which includes eating. In our culture, eating is typically not considered a sensual activity. We are taught from an early age to use a fork and spoon, and urged to be neat when we feed ourselves. "Don't eat with your fingers! Use your fork. Mind your manners!" is often a parent's first reprimand. Feeding yourself with your fingers is considered an ill-mannered or barbaric act.

In more recent times, meals are increasingly eaten alone instead of with family and friends. In American households, many meals are hastily gulped down in front of televisions, desks, and even behind steering wheels. Harried diners allow themselves to truly taste only the first few bites of their food, and then they eat as if on automatic pilot. As a result, we are cheating ourselves out of the delight that food can bring us. When we feel deprived, our brain often signals us to overeat, many times in an unconscious way.

This week, try eating as many foods as you can with your hands. Don't be afraid to get messy, and to fully experience all of the joys your meal has to offer. Strive to eat at least one meal every day without utensils.

Begin your sensory feast by taking a few cleansing breaths and sitting in silence. Practice being mindful and in the present moment. Focus only on the meal in front of you and the pleasure it brings to you. Encourage your dining partners to join you in your quest to eat with awareness. While eating with friends, instead of gossiping, share your present-moment awareness and observations.

Endeavor to notice all of your thoughts, feelings, and bodily sensations as you eat. Notice the sweetness of the first bite of apple and how it differs from the tartness of the last nibble. Savor each sensory experience as it occurs. Experiment by chewing slower or faster and noticing what happens within your body. Experiment by eating in silence. Withdraw your sense of sight and attempt to eat with your eyes closed.

For many of us, forbidden foods are often hastily devoured and followed by feelings of guilt and remorse. This week, experience a small portion of your forbidden food without guilt by eating slowly with all of your senses. Write about your experience in your journal.

Transform Your Junk Food Cravings into Healthy Desires

Craving junk food is a common occurrence for most of us trying to lose weight. At times, our compulsion to eat certain types of food can be so strong that it feels as if we are powerless. Unmet psychological needs are the primary causes of food cravings and can lead to emotional eating. Low blood sugar and fluctuating hormonal levels are two other factors that contribute to cravings, too.

When your sacral chakra is imbalanced, you are likely to use food as a mood-altering substance. Depression, boredom, stress, or simply a need for comfort, are prevalent emotional triggers for food yearnings.

Most of the time, we are not aware of our negative feelings. When painful or uncomfortable feelings arise within us, we use food to quell our anxiety. Food becomes the reliable, trusted friend that is always there for us when we need to feel better. However, the long-term consequences of emotional eating can be disastrous. Consistently indulging junk food cravings can lead to dangerous conditions such as obesity, diabetes, and heart disease. This week, learn to master your food cravings and identify the emotions that cause you to reach for unhealthy food.

Journal Away Your Cravings

This week, keep a small notebook with you at all times. When you crave a particular food, immediately stop what you are doing and take out your notebook. Before writing, take five minutes to sit quietly and pay attention to your breathing. Become aware of any sensations you feel within your body. Ask yourself these questions either silently or aloud: How are you feeling? What is your body trying to tell you? What particular food are you craving? Write these answers freely in your journal. Do not censor yourself or judge what you are writing.

What thoughts were you thinking just prior to your food craving? What thoughts are you thinking in this moment? When was the last time you ate? Is your body truly hungry or can you identify an emotional need that needs to be satisfied? For example, if you are feeling lonely, a five-minute phone call to a loved one is much more satisfying than a candy bar gulped down in guilty bites.

At the end of the week, study your notebook carefully. What patterns do you notice related to your cravings? For example, when you feel depressed, you may find yourself reaching for chocolate. Or if you are feeling overwhelmed, you may binge on potato chips. Become aware of your personal pattern. The next time you experience negative feelings such as anxiety, depression, boredom, or anger, allow yourself to fully experience them. Instead of stuffing down your feelings with food, permit your feelings to exist within you.

Your feelings are a great indicator of what you need in your life: pay close attention to them. A professional counselor is a great resource if you find yourself consistently experiencing feelings of depression or if you are unable to identify any feelings.

Now, take a look at the common foods you crave. Look at the following table, so you can transform your junk food cravings into healthy choices.

Instead of:	Indulge in:
Potato chips	2 cups plain popcorn
Ice cream	Nonfat yogurt/cottage cheese
Chocolate bar	6 small carob chips
Candy	Frozen grapes (Chapter 4)
Nachos	Chakra Salsa with Pita Squares (Chapter 1)
Cake	Organic Strawberry Banana Cupcakes (Chapter 1)
Milk shake	Mango Peach Smoothie (Chapter 2)
Peanut brittle	Solar Plexus Power Granola (Chapter 3)
Hot fudge sundae	Healthy Banana S'mores (Chapter 3)
Pie	Blueberry Wheat Muffin (Chapter 5)

Tap on Your Body to Change Your Eating Habits

Did you know that by simply tapping on certain body parts, you can create instant inner peace and curb your ravenous appetite? According to Aileen Nobles, a psychotherapist with an extensive client list that includes celebrities and political figures, you can tap on various body parts to attain any emotional state that you desire. For example, if your mouth is crying out for a bite of chocolate cake, just tap under your nose at the point between your nose and your upper lip to instantly end the craving.

This technique is known at "The Emotional Freedom Technique," or EFT. Ms. Nobles describes EFT as "emotional acupuncture without the needles." She purports that our emotions are stored in our body's energy/electromagnetic blueprint, and in our body's meridians—energetic pathways that send information throughout our entire chakra system.

Tapping on specific body parts serves as an important way to balance an otherwise-disrupted energy flow. When done properly, the results are consistent and often dramatic. This self-healing technique is easy to use and does not have any known negative side-effects. According to Ms. Nobles, once tapping is learned, it becomes a daily habit as important as brushing your teeth.

To begin tapping, use your index finger and middle finger. Tap quickly as if you were tapping to a fast-paced rendition of the tune "Jingle Bells." Tap purposefully yet gently, using about as much force as you would use to strike a letter on your computer's keyboard. Practice tapping on various chakra points to see how it feels to you.

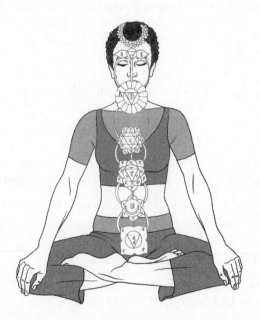

The Chakra System

Tap Away Cravings

Ms. Nobles states that in order to curb your appetite, you need to tap just under your nose at the point between your nose and your upper lip. In addition, the meridian point on your inner thigh, four finger widths above your kneecap, is also an excellent part to tap to reduce food cravings. As you tap, Ms. Nobles suggests saying the following words aloud:

"Even though I am eating to fill the emptiness inside me, I am quite wonderful anyway."

"Food is not filling me up. I would much rather eat less and feel good about myself."

"I am losing my appetite for chocolate/French fries/ice cream." (Be sure to add in any particular food craving you experience.)

Tap Away Stress

You can ease stress and enjoy feelings of inner peace by tapping on your third-eye point and acknowledging your stress. The third-eye point is located in the middle of your forehead, between your eyes and your eyebrows. Ms. Nobles suggests saying these words aloud as you tap on your third-eye center and acknowledge your stress:

"I am feeling stressed out and uptight right now."

"I really feel overwhelmed."

Ms. Nobles then states that you need to begin moving your hand toward your thymus area. Continue to verbalize your negative feelings a few more times.

As you tap on the thymus, which is the upper part of your chest cavity that sits behind your sternum, say, "Even though I am having a stressful time, I can choose to let it go and feel peace."

Continue to tap on your thymus, repeating, "I am letting it go and allowing peace to flood every cell of my body."

This week, write in your journal about your experience with tapping. How has this technique eased your stress level and your appetite?

Get Physical! Yoga for Your Sacral Chakra

The Eagle yoga posture is a great way to stimulate your sacral chakra. This posture, known as Garudasana in ancient Sanskrit, awakens your sexual organs and brings a new creative passion to your life. This pose is particularly helpful for those struggling with infertility and impotence, two common issues associated with obesity.

To begin this posture, take a few deep-cleansing breaths. Relax your body and mind. Gently close your eyes and welcome everything you are experiencing right now.

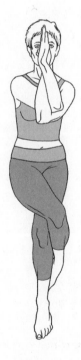

Eagle Pose

Stand with your feet together and your back straight. Extend your spine, as you imagine your vertebrae stacked one on top of the other, bone by bone.

Slowly bring your left arm under your right arm, gently folding both arms at the elbow. Release all the tension in your arms. Place your hands together, with your palms facing one another.

Gaze at a fixed point in the room at least five feet in front of you. This gaze will help you maintain your balance. Bend both of your knees. On your next inhalation, slowly cross your left leg over your right thigh or calf. If you feel steady, wrap your left foot around your right ankle.

Continue to breathe deeply. Attempt to hold this pose for five whole breaths. If you lose your balance, be gentle with yourself. Take a few deep, cleansing breaths and begin the pose again. Be sure to keep your back straight and your hips forward.

Gently release this pose. Reverse this pose on the other side of your body.

3

Your Solar Plexus Chakra

Your third chakra is known as the solar plexus chakra. It is associated with the concepts of identity and self-esteem. This energy center controls motivation, ambition, and power. Physically, the solar plexus is located near the lower ribs. It is associated with the color yellow.

Diseases associated with an unbalanced solar plexus include alcoholism, eating disorders, and digestive problems. Symptoms of a blocked third chakra include potbelly, a hard stomach, or chronic gastrointestinal issues. Weight gain and unhealthy eating habits can undermine your sense of self and your ability to have a thriving third chakra.

When people feel powerless, they may eat in a dysfunctional manner in an attempt to gain a sense of control over their lives. In the beginning, food serves to be the one area of their life they can "control." Ironically, this dysfunctional relationship with food spins out of control and begins to negatively impact other areas of their lives.

This week, you will learn to lose weight while gaining a clear sense of your life's purpose and breaking free of powerlessness and procrastination.

Let's get started by taking a look at this week's eating plan.

SOLAR PLEXUS CHAKRA SEVEN-DAY EATING PLAN

Day One

Breakfast: Banana French Toast
Midmorning Snack: 1 large grapefruit
Lunch: Piña Colada Salad
Midafternoon Snack: 1/4 cup sunflower seeds
Dinner: Lemon Spaghetti
Dessert: Heavenly Chocolate Banana Popsicle

Day Two

Breakfast: Solar Plexus Power Granola and 1 cup soy milk or skim milk
Midmorning Snack: 1/2 cup freeze-dried corn
Lunch: Water Chestnut, Onion, and Pea Salad
Midafternoon Snack: 1/2 cup Organic Corn Salsa with celery sticks
Dinner: African–Inspired Banana Chicken
Dessert: Healthy Banana S'mores

Day Three

Breakfast: Banana Split Sundae Breakfast
Midmorning Snack: 1/2 cup nonfat cottage cheese
Lunch: Yellow Pepper Power Salad
Midafternoon Snack: 1 banana and 1/4 cup walnuts
Dinner: Healthy Macaroni and Cheese
Dessert: 1/2 cup crushed pineapple

Day Four

Breakfast: Banana French Toast
Midmorning Snack: 2 cups plain popcorn
Lunch: Grapefruit Walnut Salad
Midafternoon Snack: 1 medium apple with 1 tablespoon peanut butter
Dinner: Southwestern-Style Cornbread and Chicken Casserole
Dessert: Healthy Banana S'mores

Day Five

Breakfast: Solar Plexus Power Granola with $^1/_2$ cup soy milk or skim milk

Midmorning Snack: 1 large banana

Lunch: Chakra Corn Chowder

Midafternoon Snack: Homemade Grapefruit Soda

Dinner: Hawaiian Meatballs with Butternut Squash Fries

Dessert: Pineapple Corn "Pudding"

Day Six

Breakfast: Banana French Toast

Midmorning Snack: $^1/_2$ cup nonfat yogurt

Lunch: Teriyaki Fettuccine with Watercress

Midafternoon Snack: Organic Corn Salsa with carrot sticks

Dinner: Solar Plexus Stir-Fry

Dessert: Heavenly Chocolate Banana Popsicle

Day Seven

Breakfast: Banana Split Sundae Breakfast

Midmorning Snack: 2 cups plain popcorn

Lunch: Piña Colada Salad

Midafternoon Snack: $^1/_2$ cup Organic Corn Salsa with 4 whole-wheat crackers

Dinner: Asian-Inspired Tangy Pineapple Pork

Dessert: Pineapple Corn "Pudding"

Foods That Enhance Your Solar Plexus Chakra

Fruits and vegetables that contain yellow pigments and/or skins are excellent ways to support your third energy center and your overall health.

Some fruits and vegetables with yellow skins and pigments include the following:

- Bananas
- Chestnuts
- Lemons
- Pineapples
- Rutabaga
- Spanish onions
- Vidalia onions
- Water chestnuts
- Watercress
- Yellow peppers
- Yellow squash

Solar Plexus Recipes

Here are this week's gourmet recipes that will enhance your third chakra and accelerate your weight loss.

Banana French Toast

Yield: 4 servings   *Prep time:* 6 minutes
Cook time: 6 minutes   *Serving size:* 2 small slices

3 bananas, peeled and
  sliced ½-inch thick

2 eggs

¾ cup skim milk

1 tsp. cinnamon

2 TB. brown sugar

½ tsp. vanilla extract

8 slices multigrain bread

Each serving has:

245 calories

52 g carbohydrates

3 g fat

6 g fiber

8 g protein

1. Place bananas, eggs, milk, cinnamon, brown sugar, and vanilla extract into a blender. Mix well.

2. Pour purée into shallow dish.

3. Dip each bread slice into batter for 10 seconds on each side.

4. Place bread on a nonstick skillet coated with nonstick vegetable spray. Cook over medium-high heat on both sides for about 4 minutes or until golden brown.

5. Garnish with sliced banana if desired and serve.

Hawaiian Meatballs

Yield: 6 servings   *Prep time:* 8 minutes
Cook time: 35 minutes   *Serving size:* 2 meatballs

1 lb. lean ground turkey

⅔ cup whole-wheat cracker crumbs

2 eggs

½ cup Vidalia or Spanish onion, minced

1½ tsp. salt

½ tsp. black pepper

¼ cup skim milk

1 TB. canola oil

2 TB. corn starch

½ cup brown sugar

½ cup vinegar

½ cup ketchup, organic

½ cup water

½ cup red bell pepper, finely diced

1 TB. soy sauce

10 oz. pineapple chunks in juice, drained

Each serving has:
230 calories
16 g carbohydrates
8 g fat
1 g fiber
14 g protein

1. Preheat the oven to 300°F. In a large bowl, mix ground turkey, cracker crumbs, eggs, onions, salt, and milk. Shape ground turkey mixture into small meatballs.

2. Brown meatballs in a large skillet with 1 TB. of canola oil over medium-high heat. Drain off fat and place meatballs into a large baking pan.

3. In a saucepan, combine cornstarch, brown sugar, vinegar, and ketchup. Cook over medium-high heat for about 5 minutes.

4. Gradually add water and soy sauce. Bring mixture to boil. Add red peppers and pineapple, and cook for 5 minutes. Remove the pan from heat. Pour sauce over meatballs, coating evenly.

5. Bake for 25 to 30 minutes.

6. Serve meatballs with Butternut Squash Fries.

Butternut Squash Fries

Yield: 4 servings   *Prep time:* 10 minutes
Cook time: 35 minutes   *Serving size:* 6 ounces

1 large butternut squash   Kosher salt

Each serving has:
192 calories
50 g carbohydrates
Trace fat
7 g fiber
4 g protein

1. Preheat the oven to 425°F.

2. Peel and remove seeds from butternut squash. Cut into French fries.

3. Place fries on a greased cookie sheet. Sprinkle lightly with kosher salt.

4. Bake for 35 minutes, turning halfway through bake time. Fries are ready when they are crispy and begin to brown on edges.

Lemon Spaghetti

Yield: 6 servings   *Prep time:* 8 minutes
Cook time: 25 minutes   *Serving size:* 1½ cups

½ cup freshly squeezed
lemon juice

1 TB. grated lemon zest

3 TB. extra-virgin olive oil

1 tsp. salt

½ tsp. freshly ground pepper

1 lb. whole-wheat spaghetti

½ lb. cooked chicken,
cubed into 1-inch
pieces

1 cup Parmesan cheese,
low-fat

⅓ cup fresh basil,
chopped fine

Each serving has:
450 calories
57 g carbohydrates
11 g fat
6 g fiber
28 g protein

1. To make lemon sauce: in a medium bowl, whisk together lemon juice, lemon zest, oil, salt, and pepper. Set aside.

2. Cook whole-wheat spaghetti according to directions on the package. Drain and reserve ¼ cup of water.

3. Transfer spaghetti to lemon sauce. Toss with cooked chicken, cheese, and basil. Gradually add reserved water 1 tablespoon at a time until lemon sauce evenly coats spaghetti and chicken. Serve immediately.

Banana Split Sundae Breakfast

Yield: 1 serving   *Prep time:* 10 minutes
Cook time: None   *Serving size:* 2 cups

½ cup Solar Plexus Power
Granola (recipe in this
chapter)

⅓ cup blueberries

1 large banana, sliced

8 oz. vanilla yogurt,
nonfat

¼ cup walnuts

Each serving has:
531 calories
78 g carbohydrates
10 g fat
6 g fiber
21 g protein

1. Place ⅓ granola in a tall parfait or sundae glass. Set aside. In a medium bowl, gently stir blueberries and banana slices into yogurt.

2. Place ⅓ yogurt and fruit mixture on top granola. Top with walnuts.

3. Repeat layers. Top with remaining Solar Plexus Granola. Serve immediately.

Heavenly Chocolate Banana Popsicles

Yield: 4 servings   *Prep time:* 10 minutes
Cook time: None; freeze overnight   *Serving size:* 1 popsicle

4 medium firm, ripe bananas

12 oz. semi-sweet chocolate chips (or carob chips)

¼ cup skim milk

2 TB. unsalted light butter

1 cup Solar Plexus Granola (recipe in this chapter)

Each serving has:
120 calories
22 g carbohydrates
6 g fat
1 g fiber
1 g protein

1. Peel bananas and insert a popsicle stick into one end of each banana. Be sure to leave about 2¹/₂ inches of the stick showing. Wrap loosely in waxed paper and freeze overnight, or for at least 3 hours.

2. In double boiler, melt chocolate, skim milk, and butter until smooth. Set aside. Pour 1 cup of granola on a large plate.

3. Transfer melted chocolate into tall glass. Remove bananas from freezer. Dip each banana in chocolate. Allow excess chocolate to drip off. Roll each banana in granola. Serve.

Healthy Macaroni and Cheese

Yield: 4 servings   *Prep time:* 10 minutes
Cook time: 20 minutes   *Serving size:* 1½ cups

4 cups whole-wheat rotini pasta

4 TB. extra-virgin olive oil

1 TB. flaxseed oil

½ tsp. sea salt

1 cup carrot, shredded and steamed or microwaved until crisp tender (about 3 to 5 minutes)

1 cup broccoli florets, chopped fine and steamed or micro-waved until crisp tender (about 3 to 5 minutes)

2 cups low-fat cheddar cheese, shredded

Each serving has:
510 calories
60 g carbohydrates
15 g fat
10 g fiber
30 g protein

1. Boil whole-wheat pasta according to package directions. Drain pasta, place back into the pot, and place the pot onto a hot burner, over low-medium heat.

2. Add olive oil, flaxseed oil, and salt to macaroni. Stir well to coat noodles.

3. Add shredded carrots and chopped broccoli. Mix well.

4. Add shredded cheese. Continue to stir mixture until cheese melts. Serve immediately.

Chakra Corn Chowder

Yield: 4 servings   *Prep time:* 10 minutes
Cook time: 35 minutes   *Serving size:* 1½ cups

2 TB. extra-virgin olive oil

1 cup onions, chopped fine

½ cup red bell peppers, diced small

¼ cup celery, sliced

6 cups fresh corn kernels

3 cups vegetable stock

½ cup skim milk

½ tsp. fresh rosemary, chopped fine

½ tsp. dried thyme

⅛ tsp. black pepper

1 tsp. fresh basil

Each serving has:
510 calories
60 g carbohydrates
15 g fat
10 g fiber
30 g protein

1. Pour olive oil into a large, heavy saucepan. Heat over medium heat for 2 minutes.

2. Sauté onion, red bell pepper, and celery for 5 minutes, until tender and lightly browned. Add 4 cups corn. Sauté for 5 minutes, or until corn softens.

3. Add 2 cups vegetable stock and milk. Cook for 20 minutes, or until corn can be easily mashed with a fork.

4. Transfer contents of the saucepan to a food processor or blender. Purée until smooth.

5. Return purée to the saucepan. Add rosemary, thyme, black pepper, remaining cup vegetable stock, and remaining 2 cups corn.

6. Cook for 15 minutes. Garnish with chopped basil and serve immediately.

African-Inspired Banana Chicken

Yield: 6 servings   *Prep time:* 8 minutes
Cook time: 30 minutes   *Serving size:* 6 ounces

6 bananas, ripe

1½ lb. chicken breasts,
  boned and skinned

¼ cup extra-virgin olive oil

3 tsp. cinnamon

1 tsp. paprika

Salt and pepper

Each serving has:
369 calories
29 g carbohydrates
16 g fat
4 g fiber
15 g protein

1. Preheat the oven to 350°F.

2. In a large bowl, mash bananas.

3. Arrange chicken on a baking sheet. Lightly brush each piece of chicken with olive oil.

4. Cover each piece of chicken with mashed banana. Sprinkle cinnamon and paprika over banana. Add salt and pepper to taste.

5. Bake in the oven for 30 minutes or until chicken reaches internal temperature of 165°F. Serve.

Pineapple Corn "Pudding"

Yield: 8 servings   *Prep time:* 5 minutes
Cook time: None; refrigerate overnight   *Serving size:* 6 ounces

14 oz. crushed pineapple, drained

12 oz. whole-kernel corn, drained

¼ cup mayonnaise, low-fat

1 TB. organic honey

1 tsp. cinnamon

Each serving has:
95 calories
12 g carbohydrates
6 g fat
Trace fiber
Trace protein

1. In a large bowl, mix pineapple and corn.

2. Add mayonnaise, honey, and cinnamon. Mix well. Refrigerate overnight. Place 6 ounces of pudding into individual cups and serve.

Grapefruit Walnut Salad

Yield: 4 servings   *Prep time:* 10 minutes
Cook time: None   *Serving size:* 2 cups

2 cups spinach leaves

1 pink grapefruit, peeled and membranes removed

2 avocados, peeled and seeded, sliced into 2-inch pieces

¼ cup Gorgonzola cheese, crumbled

½ cup walnuts, chopped

¼ cup honey mustard salad dressing, fat-free

Each serving has:
352 calories
19 g carbohydrates
17 g fat
4 g fiber
9 g protein

1. Spread spinach on a large round platter.

2. Place grapefruit and avocado on top spinach.

3. Sprinkle salad with Gorgonzola cheese and walnuts. Drizzle with honey mustard dressing. Serve family-style.

Teriyaki Fettuccine with Watercress

Yield: 4 servings   *Prep time:* 10 minutes
Cook time: 20 minutes   *Serving size:* 2 cups

1 lb. whole-wheat fettuccine pasta

1 TB. extra-virgin olive oil

12 crimini mushrooms, sliced thin

Salt and pepper

1 cup watercress, washed and dried, trimmed, cut into 2-inch pieces

1½ cups vegetable stock

¼ cup teriyaki sauce

1 TB. cornstarch

¼ cup cold water

1 TB. light butter

1 lb. whole-wheat fettuccine pasta, cooked

Each serving has:
398 calories
40 g carbohydrates
8 g fat
4 g fiber
5 g protein

1. Heat a skillet over medium-high heat with olive oil.

2. Add mushrooms. Sauté for 5 minutes until brown and tender. Season with salt and pepper.

3. Add watercress. Sauté for 2 minutes. Gradually add vegetable stock and teriyaki sauce, and stir mixture.

4. In a small bowl, dissolve cornstarch into cold water, and stir well. Pour cornstarch mixture into the skillet. Bring mixture to rapid boil. Sauce will thicken as it boils. Add butter to mixture prior to serving to give sauce a glossy finish.

5. Toss sauce with hot pasta. Serve.

Healthy Banana S'mores

Yield: 6 servings   *Prep time:* 5 minutes
Cook time: 2 minutes   *Serving size:* 1 cookie

6 low-fat graham crackers, broken in half

1½ oz. dark chocolate, broken into small pieces

1 banana, sliced thin

½ cup fresh strawberries, sliced

Each serving has:
81 calories
14 g carbohydrates
3 g fat
1 g fiber
1 g protein

1. Preheat the broiler.

2. Place graham cracker halves on a baking sheet. Top each half with 2 dark chocolate pieces.

3. Place 4 banana slices and 2 slices strawberries on top chocolate pieces.

4. Broil for 2 minutes. Serve immediately.

Water Chestnut, Onion, and Pea Salad

Yield: 4 servings   *Prep time:* 10 minutes
Cook time: None   *Serving size:* 1 cup

1 can water chestnuts, canned, sliced

1 cup sweet peas

1 cup diced red onion

¼ cup peanuts, chopped

2 TB. sesame oil

1 tsp. curry powder

1 TB. low-fat peanut butter

1 TB. sesame seeds

1 TB. soy sauce

Pinch ground ginger

1 head bok choy, chopped

Each serving has:
400 calories
24 g carbohydrates
19 g fat
6 g fiber
20 g protein

1. Combine water chestnuts, peas, onions, and peanuts in a large bowl.

2. In a separate bowl mix sesame oil, curry powder, peanut butter, sesame seeds, soy sauce, and ginger.

3. Combine sesame mixture with water chestnut mixture and gently toss. Allow salad to stand for 15 minutes.

4. Serve water chestnut mixture on bed of bok choy.

Asian-Inspired Tangy Pineapple Pork

Yield: 6 servings   *Prep time:* 10 minutes
Cook time: 45 minutes   *Serving size:* 1 pork chop

6 (8 oz.) lean pork chops

6 TB. light soy sauce

6 TB. teriyaki sauce

2 TB. fresh ginger chopped

4 TB. sesame oil

Dash white pepper

1 (10 oz.) can pineapple chunks in juice

¼ cup red bell pepper, diced small

Each serving has:

94 calories

5 g carbohydrates

8 g fat

1 g fiber

1 g protein

1. Preheat the oven to 400°F.

2. Rinse and dry each pork chop. Place on a greased 9×8-inch baking pan.

3. In a medium bowl, combine soy sauce, teriyaki sauce, ginger, sesame oil, and white pepper. Pour over pork.

4. Pour pineapples and juice over pork mixture. Sprinkle with red peppers.

5. Bake, uncovered, for 40 to 45 minutes or until pork reaches internal temperature of 160°F.

Solar Plexus Power Granola

Yield: 9 servings   *Prep time:* 10 minutes
Cook time: 30 minutes   *Serving size:* 1 cup

4 cups cooked rolled oats

1 cup wheat germ

¼ cup walnuts, chopped fine

¼ cup almonds, chopped fine

½ cup sesame seeds

1 tsp. cinnamon

1 tsp. salt

¼ cup sugar

⅔ cup maple syrup

⅓ cup extra-virgin olive oil

⅓ cup water

Each serving has:
294 calories
27 g carbohydrates
18 g fat
5 g fiber
9 g protein

1. Preheat the oven to 400°F.

2. In a large bowl, combine oats, wheat germ, walnuts, almonds, sesame seeds, cinnamon, salt, and sugar. Make a well in mixture. Gradually stir in maple syrup, olive oil, and water. Coat dry ingredients thoroughly.

3. Spread mixture evenly onto a large cookie sheet that is coated with nonstick vegetable cooking spray. Bake for 20 minutes or until mixture is brown and lightly toasted, stirring halfway through baking time.

4. Allow mixture to cool for 30 minutes. Serve, or store in an airtight container.

Piña Colada Salad

Yield: 8 servings   *Prep time:* 10 minutes
Cook time: None; refrigerate overnight   *Serving size:* 1 cup

1 small pineapple, cubed

2 cups strawberries, halved

1 small papaya, cubed

1 cup nonfat vanilla yogurt

⅛ tsp. ground cinnamon

¼ cup coconut, flaked

2 kiwifruit, peeled and sliced

Each serving has:
101 calories
22 g carbohydrates
1 g fat
3 g fiber
2 g protein

1. In a large bowl, combine pineapple, strawberries, and papaya.

2. In a small bowl, stir together yogurt, cinnamon, and coconut. Pour mixture over fruit. Toss well.

3. Cover salad and chill overnight.

4. Just prior to serving, add kiwi slices and gently combine.

Yellow Pepper Power Salad

Yield: 8 servings   *Prep time:* 10 minutes
Cook time: None   *Serving size:* 1 cup

⅓ cup Balsamic vinegar

3 TB. extra-virgin olive oil

1 large Vidalia or Spanish onion, sliced thin

1 tsp. turmeric

1 tsp. cumin

Sea salt and pepper

2 lb. green beans, trimmed and halved crosswise

1 TB. freshly chopped basil

2 lb. yellow bell peppers, sliced ½-inch thick

Each serving has:
108 calories
15 g carbohydrates
5 g fat
5 g fiber
3 g protein

1. In a large bowl, whisk together Balsamic vinegar and oil. Toss in Vidalia onion. Add turmeric and cumin. Season to taste with sea salt and pepper. Set aside.

2. In a large pot of boiling water, cook green beans 10 minutes or until slightly tender. Drain in a colander and rinse with cold water. Pat dry.

3. Add green beans, chopped basil, and yellow peppers to the large bowl with vinegar and onion mixture. Toss well. Serve.

Southwestern-Style Cornbread and Chicken Casserole

Yield: 6 servings   *Prep time:* 10 minutes
Cook time: 30 minutes   *Serving size:* 1 slice

4 TB. extra-virgin olive oil

1 Vidalia or Spanish onion, chopped fine

¼ cup red bell pepper, chopped fine

¼ cup green pepper, chopped fine

2 cups cooked chicken, cubed

1 cup sour cream, fat-free

½ tsp. thyme

¼ tsp. sage

Dash cayenne

1 cup cheddar cheese, grated, divided

1 cup yellow cornmeal, whole-grain

1½ tsp. baking powder

¼ tsp. salt

½ cup whole-wheat flour

⅓ cup skim milk

1 egg, slightly beaten

17 oz. creamed corn

Each serving has:
450 calories
44 g carbohydrates
16 g fat
5 g fiber
26 g protein

1. In a large skillet, heat olive oil over medium-high heat. Add onion, red peppers, and green peppers. Cook 5 minutes or until vegetables are slightly tender.

2. Add cooked chicken, sour cream, thyme, sage, cayenne, and ½ cup cheddar cheese. Cook over low heat for 2 minutes. Remove the pan from heat and set aside.

3. Grease a large baking pan (9×9×2-inch). Preheat the oven to 425°F.

4. In a large bowl, combine cornmeal, baking powder, salt, whole-wheat flour, milk, egg, and creamed corn. Mix well. Pour into the greased baking pan.

5. Top with chicken mixture. Bake for 15 minutes. Top with remaining cheddar cheese.

6. Continue baking for 15 minutes or until lightly browned on top.

7. Let stand for 10 minutes before cutting and serving.

Homemade Grapefruit Soda

Yield: 4 servings   *Prep time:* 15 minutes
Cook time: None   *Serving size:* 1 cup

1½ cups fresh-squeezed
    grapefruit juice
3 TB. organic honey

½ tsp. nutmeg
2 cinnamon sticks
24 oz. seltzer water

Each serving has:
102 calories
27 g carbohydrates
Trace fat
4 g fiber
1 g protein

1. In a medium saucepan, combine grapefruit juice, honey, nutmeg, and cinnamon sticks.

2. Bring to boil, then immediately reduce heat.

3. Allow syrupy mixture to simmer uncovered for 5 minutes.

4. Discard cinnamon sticks, and allow syrup to cool for 7 minutes.

5. Fill 4 (8-oz.) glasses with ice.

6. Add ⅓ cup grapefruit syrup to each glass. Fill the glasses to top with seltzer water. Gently stir. Serve.

Organic Corn Salsa

Yield: 4 servings   *Prep time:* 10 minutes
Cook time: None; refrigerate 3 hours   *Serving size:* ⅓ cup

1 cup organic corn kernels

2 medium tomatoes, chopped

1 small Vidalia or Spanish onion, chopped fine

½ cup fresh cilantro, minced

2 TB. green peppers, chopped fine

1 TB. red bell pepper, chopped fine

1 tsp. jalapeño pepper, seeded and minced

¼ tsp. salt

Dash pepper

Each serving has:
59 calories
14 g carbohydrates
Trace fat
2 g fiber
2 g protein

1. Combine corn, tomatoes, onion, cilantro, green and red bell peppers, jalapeños, salt, and pepper in a bowl.

2. Refrigerate for at least 3 hours before serving. Serve with whole-wheat crackers, carrots, and sliced green and red peppers.

Solar Plexus Stir-Fry

Yield: 4 servings   *Prep time:* 10 minutes
Cook time: 15 minutes   *Serving size:* ⅓ cup

2 TB. plus 2 tsp. sunflower oil

3 cloves garlic, minced

1 lb. chicken, boned and skinned and cut into 2-inch pieces

Salt and pepper

3 heads broccoli, chopped coarse

1 cup carrots, peeled and chopped

1 small Vidalia onion, chopped thin

16 oz. mushroom caps

¼ cup teriyaki sauce

4 cups hot, cooked brown rice

Each serving has:
502 calories
50 g carbohydrates
16 fat
13 g fiber
31 g protein

1. In a large skillet, heat 2 tablespoons sunflower oil over medium-high heat. Add garlic to the pan. Sauté for 3 minutes, or until golden.

2. Add chicken pieces to the pan. Season with salt and pepper. Stir-fry chicken on all sides for 5 minutes until chicken is lightly browned. Remove chicken and garlic from the pan and set aside

3. Add 2 additional teaspoons sunflower oil to the pan, over medium-high heat. Add broccoli, carrots, onions, and mushrooms. Stir-fry for 6 minutes or until vegetables are tender.

4. Return chicken and garlic to the pan. Add teriyaki sauce. Stir-fry for another 2 minutes, until chicken reaches internal temperature of 165°F.

5. Serve chicken mixture over brown rice.

Exercises to Balance Your Solar Plexus Chakra

Let's get started with some personal-growth exercises that will balance your third energy center.

Finish Your Old Business and Reclaim Your Power!

Most of us have projects or chores that we've left half done or have abandoned altogether. In modern life, it seems as if there is never enough time to accomplish all we set out to do. We start a project with the best of intentions, only to get sidetracked to meet the demands of our family or work.

Our subconscious mind remains aware of all of these tasks that we started but never completed. Although we may not consciously think about these abandoned projects daily, our subconscious mind never forgets about them. Gradually, our old, unfinished business erodes our self-esteem and sense of personal power.

Unworthiness erodes our third energy center and packs the pounds on our waistline. In an effort to avoid these negative emotions, many people use food to quiet their subconscious minds and stuff their feelings.

Journal Exercise: Handling Your Business

This week, vow to complete the unfinished business that drains your energy and sabotages your weight-loss goals.

Relax; resist the temptation to skip this exercise. Finishing old business does not mean that you have to stay up all night completing that boring correspondence course or organizing your CD collection.

Simply take out your journal and a pen. Before beginning this activity, sit quietly and take a few deep, cleansing breaths. Next, write down all of the projects that you started but never completed. In your list, you also may include things you know you need to do but have not yet taken action on. After you feel you've exhausted every possible piece of unfinished business, take a moment to sit in silence and review your items.

Now think of all the unfinished relationship business that exists in your life. If you are having difficulty thinking of items for your list, imagine that you only had a month left to live to get your affairs in order. After you have completed both lists, carefully read them to make sure you have not forgotten anything or anyone. You now have an opportunity to complete the business and increase your self-esteem. Look at each item and decide how you want to deal with it. You have four choices that you can take to remedy these undone items and create a sense of inner peace for yourself. You can choose to finish the business now, complete it by a specific date, delegate it, or forget about it entirely:

- **Finish old business right now**   Completing old business right in the moment is a quick and effective way to reclaim your power. For example, you could pick up the phone right now and tell your estranged daughter that you will always love her unconditionally even if you do not like her behavior.

- **Set a date to handle your business**   Perhaps you do not have the time, energy, or economic resources to complete your old business right now. If this is the case, set a target date in the near future by which you can accomplish your goal.

- **Delegate your old business**   Many times, we avoid completing items because we find the task exceedingly unpleasant, or we lack the skills to get the job done right. Make a decision today to stop torturing yourself and to call a professional or enlist the help of a trusted friend.

Decide which items on your list you want to give up entirely. Cross these items off your list in indelible ink. Or you may choose to write down these items on a separate sheet of paper and safely burn or bury them.

End Procrastination in Just Seven Minutes

Procrastination is a self-defeating habit that makes us feel stuck, paralyzed by fear and indecision. Chronic procrastination is a hallmark of a blocked third chakra. Many people procrastinate about starting a diet or beginning an exercise plan. It is very easy to say that you will start a diet tomorrow. The trouble is that tomorrow never comes, but your feelings of powerlessness, hopelessness, and anxiety always stay with you.

There is hope. The first step to ending procrastination forever is to focus precisely on what you have been procrastinating about. Make a list of all the things you have been avoiding. This task should be simple. You can look at your "Unfinished Business Exercise" to help point you to the areas in your life where you have been procrastinating.

Choose one item you procrastinate about that causes you the most pain. Perhaps you chronically procrastinate about exercise, and you long to have a lean, sculpted physique. Make a decision to stop procrastinating about exercise today, and get started on your dream body.

Obtain a kitchen timer or similar timekeeping device, and set it for seven minutes. Exercise until the timer goes off. I guarantee that the first three minutes will be the most difficult. Your mind and body will urge you to quit. Observe how something magical happens around minute number four. You feel yourself start to get into the flow. Fully experience this feeling of flow and be aware that you are accomplishing this task.

Use the seven-minute timer to jump-start any area of your life in which you find yourself procrastinating.

Think Thin and Be Thin

This week, create a new, healthy body just by using the powers of your mind. Thinking negative thoughts about your body usually leads to negative emotions. When you experience these negative emotions, negative behaviors such as overeating often ensue. This week you will learn how to break the negative thought, feeling, and behavior cycle and transform your life forever.

Changing your thoughts can seem like an extremely difficult process. It may seem as if you have no control over your thoughts. "But these thoughts just happen!" one client exclaimed. "It's like I am having an endless conversation with myself, and it's all bad. I find fault with everything I do. I constantly beat myself up!" Know that you have the power to transform these negative thoughts into positive ones.

This week, imagine that you are the thin person you have always wanted to be. You have reached your goal weight and feel happy and peaceful. What kinds of thoughts do you think, now that you are thin? How do you view yourself and the world around you? For example, when the invitation for your class reunion arrives in the mail, you now think, "Great! Now I get my chance to connect with my old friends and show off my new, sexy body," instead of, "I have nothing to wear, and I am so ashamed of how I let myself go." How do you feel now that you are thin? Do you feel happier and lighter? How has your behavior changed now that you have reached your goal weight? How do you move your body now that you are thin? Walk with newfound confidence and hold your head up high. Pay attention to how the thin people you admire move, speak, and behave. Try to emulate their actions and conduct. How do you use your voice now that you are thin? Is your voice more authoritative or bubbly? Are you more animated? Write about your experiences in your journal.

Journal Exercise: Write Off Those Negative Thoughts

This week, make a list of your most common negative thoughts. Next to each thought, write about the specific emotions and feelings that the thought causes you to experience. Then, write about how these thoughts and feelings trigger negative behaviors such as overeating, gossiping, or compulsive shopping. What have you learned about yourself? How can you change these negative thoughts and transform yourself to a person who "thinks thin"?

Clear Clutter and Shed Extra Pounds

Living in a cluttered environment is stressful. It drains your emotional and physical energy. Messy, disorganized homes and offices often cause irritability, worry, and depression. The lack of focus and clarity you feel from living in a cluttered environment is a huge trigger for emotional eating. Weight gain and inner turmoil often directly accompany clutter and disorganization. One of the fastest ways to clear your solar plexus chakra and reclaim your personal power is to manage your clutter effectively. Clearing clutter will help you focus on your weight-loss goals and shed more pounds rapidly.

Journal Exercise: Write Off Your Clutter

This week, write about how your clutter affects you. With your journal in hand, take a tour of your office, car, and home. Sit in each room and write about how the disorganization makes you feel. Imagine your life free of the negative effects of the clutter. Picture everything in your home neatly catalogued and organized. Write about your experiences in your journal.

Tackle Your Clutter

Tackling your clutter involves courage and hard work. However, this process is so emotionally freeing that it is well worth the effort. Set aside a weekend to begin your de-cluttering process. If you feel particularly attached to your possessions, enlist the help of a trusted friend or loved one. Your mission is to do one of the following with your clutter:

- Throw away your clutter.
- Donate your clutter.
- Fix or mend your broken clutter.
- Find a home for your clutter.
- Box and label your clutter.

The book *Ask and It is Given* by Esther and Jerry Hicks contains an exercise titled: The Process of Clearing Clutter for Clarity. I highly recommend this book and this specific exercise.

Meditation to Increase Personal Power

Assume a seated posture on the floor or in a chair. Gently close your eyes. Allow a feeling of total relaxation and tranquility to wash over your entire body.

Take a few deep, cleansing breaths. Pay attention to your breathing. Feel the air enter your lungs as you inhale. Feel the air leave your lungs as you exhale.

Be here in this moment. Do not attempt to change or alter anything. Accept everything how it is.

Breathe in good health and power. Take a slow, deep breath in as you imagine inhaling a sense of good health and personal power.

Breathe out negativity and stress. Slowly exhale as you imagine releasing your negativity and stress to the universe.

Breathe in joy. Again, take a slow, deep breath. Gently smile as you draw in a sense of you and happiness.

Breathe out anger. Slowly release any anger or tension you feel in your body.

Visualize a bright white light in your solar plexus region. This is a healing light that fills the area around your lower ribs and stomach.

With each breath you take, imagine this light spreading throughout your entire body. Focus on each area of your body for a few minutes as you continue to breathe deeply. Pay attention to any problem areas in your body that need special attention or healing. Take as much time as you need focusing on this white, healing light.

At the end of the meditation, offer thanks for your newfound sense of personal power and peace.

Get Physical! Reclaim Your Power Through Yoga

Bow pose, known as Dhanurasana in ancient Sanskrit, is a yoga posture that stimulates your solar plexus chakra and awakens your inner sense of personal power.

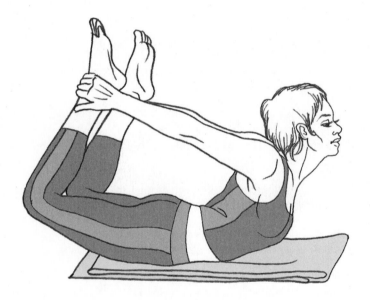

Bow Pose

Lie on your stomach. It is especially important to assume this pose on an empty stomach as it places pressure on your abdominal area. Allow your chin to gently rest on the floor. Place your legs approximately 12 inches apart.

On your next inhalation, bend both knees, and bring your heels toward the back of your thighs. Reach back with your hands and grab your ankles, one ankle at a time. Exhale.

Take a deep breath. As you exhale, gently press your pelvis into the floor as you engage your core abdominal muscles.

On your next inhalation, slowly raise your head and feet simultaneously. If you are able to, carefully lift your knees and thighs off the floor, one body part at a time. If you have a history of back or neck problems, please consult your doctor before assuming this posture. Draw your shoulder blades close together. Exhale deeply.

Gently rock back and forth in this pose for five complete breaths. Focus on your breath and your solar plexus region.

When you are ready to release the pose, begin by releasing your hands. Slowly lower and straighten your legs. Gently roll over onto your back, and deeply relax as you allow your whole body to sink into the floor. Feel a sense of personal power and peace in your solar plexus region.

4

Your Heart Chakra

Above the solar plexus is the fourth chakra, otherwise known as the heart chakra. The heart chakra is behind the sternum, and is physically associated with the thymus gland and the heart. It is represented by the color green and the energy of love. Your heart chakra connects your three lower chakras to your three upper chakras.

People with a blocked fourth chakra may struggle with depression, romantic rejection, or jealously. Isolation and loneliness may be constant companions for those with heart chakra issues.

Because we often use food as a substitute for love, the fourth chakra can cause significant weight gain when it is not functioning properly. When we hunger for love and do not receive the love we desire, we turn to food in an effort to meet our needs. In order to achieve permanent weight loss and bliss, the heart chakra must be brought back into alignment. When the heart center is dysfunctional, a person may have difficulty experiencing empathy or compassion for themselves or others.

Wear green clothing and gemstones in an effort to stimulate your heart center this week. This week you will learn how to lose weight while opening your heart to experience true compassion, kindheartedness, and devotion toward yourself and others.

Let's get started by taking a look at this week's eating plan.

HEART CHAKRA SEVEN-DAY EATING PLAN

Day One

Breakfast: Baked Eggs Florentine Casserole

Midmorning Snack: 1 large green apple with 1 tablespoon of peanut butter

Lunch: Go Green Earth Salad

Midafternoon Snack: 1/4 cup Chakra Avocado Dip with carrot and celery sticks

Dinner: Cheesy Spinach Mini-Pies

Dessert: Pear Yogurt Bread

Day Two

Breakfast: Grape and Cream Cheese Breakfast Tostada

Midmorning Snack: 10 frozen grapes

Lunch: Spicy Chicken and Avocado Lettuce Wraps

Midafternoon Snack: 1 large pear

Dinner: Asparagus, Artichoke, and Crab Quiche

Dessert: 1 slice honeydew melon

Day Three

Breakfast: Asparagus Egg-White Omelet

Midmorning Snack: 1/2 cup nonfat cottage cheese and 1 kiwi

Lunch: Go Green Earth Salad

Midafternoon Snack: 1 dill pickle

Dinner: Spinach and Turkey Wrap

Dessert: Granny Smith Apple Slaw

Day Four

Breakfast: Baked Eggs Florentine Casserole

Midmorning Snack: 1 large pear

Lunch: Toasted Chicken and Grape Grinder

Midafternoon Snack: 10 celery sticks with nonfat cream cheese

Dinner: Spicy Chicken and Avocado Lettuce Wraps

Dessert: Sliced pears topped with low-fat yogurt and chopped walnuts

Day Five

Breakfast: Baked Eggs Florentine Casserole

Midmorning Snack: 1 kiwi

Lunch: Cheesy Spinach Mini-Pies

Midafternoon Snack: Carrot sticks with Chakra Avocado Dip

Dinner: Avocado Cucumber Salad

Dessert: Granny Smith Apple Slaw

Day Six

Breakfast: Asparagus Egg-White Omelet

Midmorning Snack: $1/2$ cup raw cashew nuts

Lunch: Celery and Apple Salad

Midafternoon Snack: 1 cup steamed broccoli

Dinner: Asparagus, Artichoke, and Crab Quiche

Dessert: Frozen Grape Delight

Day Seven

Breakfast: Baked Eggs Florentine Casserole

Midmorning Snack: 1 large green apple with 1 tablespoon peanut butter

Lunch: Broccoli Soba Noodles

Midafternoon Snack: Avocado Cucumber Salad

Dinner: Spinach Pear Salad with Pear Vinaigrette and Walnuts

Dessert: Pear Yogurt Bread

Foods That Enhance Your Heart Chakra

Fruits and vegetables that contain green pigments and/or skins are excellent ways to support your fourth energy center and your overall health.

Some fruits and vegetables with green skins and pigments include the following:

- Artichokes
- Asparagus
- Avocados
- Broccoli
- Brussels sprouts
- Cabbage
- Celery
- Cucumbers
- Edamame
- Green apples
- Green grapes
- Green peppers
- Honeydew melon
- Kiwifruit
- Lettuce
- Limes
- Pears
- Peas
- Spinach
- Zucchini

Heart Chakra Recipes

Here are this week's gourmet recipes that will enhance your fourth chakra and accelerate weight loss.

Cheesy Spinach Mini-Pies

Yield: 12 servings   *Prep time:* 15 minutes
Cook time: 30 minutes   *Serving size:* 1 mini-pie

2 sheets phyllo dough

2 tsp. canola oil, cooking spray

3 cups frozen spinach chopped

4 TB. fresh garlic

Dash kosher salt

Dash white pepper

1½ cups feta cheese, crumbled

1 whole egg, beaten

½ cup water

12 oz. Parmesan cheese, grated

Each serving has:
244 calories
6 g carbohydrates
16 g fat
2 g fiber
18 g protein

1. Preheat the oven to 325°F. Remove phyllo dough from the freezer and place sheets on a clean, dry surface to thaw.

2. Place a large skillet over medium-high heat. Lightly spray with cooking spray.

3. Cook spinach and garlic about 2 to 3 minutes. Season with salt and white pepper.

4. Remove from heat and let cool for 5 minutes. Add feta.

5. Using a large cup, knife, or cookie cutter, cut out portions of phyllo dough ¹/₂-inch larger than the opening in the muffin pan.

6. Using a floured rolling pin, lightly roll out circle portions of phyllo dough.

7. Whisk together egg and water. Brush both sides of dough with egg mixture.

8. Lightly spray each muffin cup with cooking spray. Push dough portion into each muffin cup, making sure about ¹/₄ inch overlaps rim of cup.

9. Fill each cup with spinach and feta mixture. Sprinkle 2 tablespoons of Parmesan cheese on top of each cup.

10. Place the muffin pan into center of the oven. Bake for 25 to 30 minutes, or until dough and cheese have browned.

11. Remove from the oven and let stand for 5 minutes. Carefully remove mini-pies from the muffin pan and serve.

Frozen Grape Delight

Yield: 4 servings   *Prep time:* 5 minutes
Cook time: None; freeze overnight   *Serving size:* Approximately 16 grapes

1 large bunch green seed-
  less grapes

1 tsp. confectioner's
  sugar

Each serving has:
27 calories
7 g carbohydrates
Trace fat
1 g fiber
Trace protein

1. Place bunch of grapes in a large freezer bag and seal. Freeze overnight.

2. Prior to serving, lightly sprinkle grapes with confectioner's sugar.

Asparagus Egg-White Omelet

Yield: 1 serving   *Prep time:* 10 minutes
Cook time: 5 minutes   *Serving size:* 1 omelet

2 TB. asparagus, diced fine

2 TB. fresh mushrooms, diced fine

4 egg whites

2 TB. low-fat cheddar cheese, shredded

Each serving has:
97 calories
3 g carbohydrates
1 g fat
1 g fiber
18 g protein

1. Combine asparagus and mushrooms in a small bowl.

2. Whisk egg whites.

3. Spray a skillet with nonstick vegetable spray. Heat on the stove on medium-high heat. Cook vegetable mixture for 1 to 2 minutes. Set aside.

4. Pour egg whites into the skillet. Cook for approximately 4 minutes, stirring constantly. Add vegetable mixture and sprinkle with cheese. Cook for an additional minute or until cheese is melted. Fold omelet onto a plate and serve immediately.

Avocado Cucumber Salad

Yield: 8 servings   *Prep time:* 15 minutes
Cook time: None   *Serving size:* 1¹/₂ cups

14 oz. iceberg lettuce,
  washed and patted dry

2 large avocados, peeled
  and chopped

1 large cucumber, peeled
  and sliced

1 cup carrot, shredded

1 pint grape tomatoes,
  halved

½ cup almonds, chopped

½ cup extra-virgin olive
  oil

¼ cup Balsamic vinegar

1 package dry Italian
  dressing mix

4 oz. crumbled feta
  cheese

Each serving has:
308 calories
10 g carbohydrates
19 g fat
4 g fiber
6 g protein

1. In a large bowl, combine lettuce, avocado, cucumber, carrots, grape
   tomatoes, and almonds. Set aside.

2. In a medium bowl, whisk together olive oil, Balsamic vinegar, and
   package of dry Italian dressing mix. Add crumbled feta.

3. Drizzle dressing over vegetables. Toss gently to coat.

Spinach and Turkey Wraps with Cranberry Mayo

Yield: 4 servings   *Prep time:* 45 minutes
Cook time: None   *Serving size:* 1 wrap

2 oz. Craisins (dried, sweet
  cranberries)
1 cup water
1 cup mayonnaise, fat-free
1 tsp. onion powder
Dash salt

Dash white pepper
4 whole-wheat tortillas,
  96 percent fat-free
1 oz. fresh spinach,
  cleaned
1 lb. turkey, sliced

Each serving has:
380 calories
50 g carbohydrates
9 g fat
3 g fiber
22 g protein

1. Place dried, sweet cranberries in 1 cup water to soften for about half
   an hour. Remove cranberries from the water bowl and pat dry with a
   paper towel.

2. Chop cranberries coarsely with a knife or food processor. Place in a
   medium bowl.

3. Add mayonnaise, onion powder, salt, and pepper to the medium bowl.
   Stir well.

4. Lay tortillas flat and spread evenly with cranberry mayo.

5. Place spinach and turkey on one edge of each tortilla.

6. Fold smaller edge over turkey, and roll. When halfway through wrapping, fold edges inward to seal wrap. Complete roll so all ingredients
   are tightly inside tortilla.

Hearty Chakra Guacamole with Whole-Wheat Pita Squares

Yield: 8 servings   *Prep time:* 15 minutes
Cook time: None; refrigerate overnight   *Serving size:* 1/2 cup

2 medium avocados, peeled and mashed

1 TB. lemon juice

1 medium onion, minced

1 large tomato, peeled and chopped fine

1/2 tsp. chili powder

1/2 tsp. garlic, minced

Hot sauce, to taste

Salt and pepper

Each serving has:
91 calories
6 g carbohydrates
5 g fat
2 g fiber
1 g protein

1. In a large bowl, combine avocados, lemon juice, onion, tomatoes, chili powder, and garlic. Add hot sauce, salt, and pepper to taste.

2. Mix well. Cover the bowl and chill overnight in the refrigerator.

3. Serve with whole-wheat pita bread cut into squares, red bell pepper strips, carrot sticks, and celery sticks.

Spicy Chicken and Avocado Lettuce Wraps

Yield: 4 servings   *Prep time:* 15 minutes
Cook time: None   *Serving size:* 1 wrap

2½ oz. cellophane noodles

¼ cup low-sodium soy
sauce

1 tsp. fresh ginger, grated

¼ cup fresh cilantro

1 TB. chile paste

2 tsp. dark sesame oil

2 cups cooked chicken,
shredded

12 large Boston lettuce
leaves

1 large avocado, sliced

Each serving has:
300 calories
21 g carbohydrates
13 g fat
2 g fiber
24 g protein

1. Soak cellophane noodles in boiling water for 5 minutes. Drain, rinse, and chop noodles.

2. In a large bowl, whisk together soy sauce, ginger, cilantro, chile paste, and sesame oil.

3. Add noodles and cooked chicken to soy sauce mixture. Toss well.

4. Spoon chicken mixture down center of each Boston lettuce leaf. Top with avocado slices and wrap. Serve.

Asparagus, Artichoke, and Crab Quiche

Yield: 8 servings   *Prep time:* 10 minutes
Cook time: 25 minutes   *Serving size:* 1 slice

1 refrigerated piecrust

3 eggs

¼ cup asparagus, trimmed and cut into ½-inch pieces

¼ cup artichoke hearts, chopped

¼ cup red bell pepper, diced fine

¼ cup Vidalia onion, chopped fine

1 cup skim milk

1 cup low-fat Swiss cheese, cubed

8 oz. low-fat cream cheese, softened and cut into 2-inch squares

½ lb. crabmeat, picked clean

1 tsp. Old Bay Seafood seasoning

Each serving has:
281 calories
18 g carbohydrates
16 g fat
1 g fiber
15 g protein

1. Preheat the oven to 350°F. Line a pie plate with piecrust.

2. In a large bowl, whisk eggs.

3. Gradually add asparagus, artichoke hearts, red bell peppers, onion, milk, cheese, and cream cheese to bowl. Stir thoroughly.

4. Gently fold crabmeat into mixture. Pour mixture into the pie plate.

5. Bake for 45 minutes to 1 hour, or until knife inserted into the center comes out clean. Remove from the oven. Sprinkle quiche with Old Bay seasoning. Serve.

Toasted Chicken and Grape Grinder

Yield: 4 servings   *Prep time:* 10 minutes
Cook time: 10 minutes   *Serving size:* 1 sandwich

1 cup green seedless grapes, chopped coarse

⅓ cup fresh basil, chopped

¼ cup Vidalia onion, chopped

1 clove garlic, minced

2 TB. cilantro, chopped

⅓ cup Italian salad dressing, low-calorie

1 cup low-fat Mozzarella cheese

1 loaf whole-wheat bread, sliced in half horizontally

¾ lb. cooked chicken

Each serving has:
248 calories
9 g carbohydrates
10 g fat
2 g fiber
36 g protein

1. In a large bowl, combine grapes, basil, onion, garlic, cilantro, and Italian dressing.

2. Sprinkle ½ cup Mozzarella cheese on bottom half whole-wheat loaf. Top cheese with chicken. Top chicken with grape mixture. Sprinkle remaining cheese over top grape mixture.

3. Wrap bread loaf in heavy-duty foil. Grill over medium heat for 6 minutes. Turn over, and grill for additional 6 minutes.

4. Carefully remove foil and unwrap sandwich. Cut into 4 portions. Serve.

Grape and Cream Cheese Breakfast Tostada

Yield: 1 serving   *Prep time:* 5 minutes
Cook time: 12 minutes   *Serving size:* 1 sandwich

1 whole-wheat tortilla,
  6-inch
2 TB. nonfat cream cheese
½ cup green seedless
  grapes

1 tsp. cinnamon
1 TB. golden seedless
  raisins

Each serving has:
259 calories
52 g carbohydrates
3 g fat
4 g fiber
9 g protein

1. Preheat the oven to 375°F. Place tortilla on a greased baking sheet.

2. Spread cream cheese on tortilla. Gently place grapes on top cream cheese.

3. Sprinkle with cinnamon, and top with raisins. Fold tortilla in half or leave open-faced, if desired.

4. Bake for 12 to 15 minutes until crispy.

5. Slice in quarters and serve.

Go Green Earth Salad

Yield: 6 servings   *Prep time:* 10 minutes
Cook time: None   *Serving size:* 6 ounces

1½ lb. fresh baby spinach, washed and dried, torn into pieces

2 medium avocados, diced into 2-inch pieces

½ cup green olives, pitted and sliced thin

½ cup red onion, sliced thin

1 medium cucumber, sliced thin

1 cup mandarin oranges, drained and diced

1 TB. lime juice

¼ cup Balsamic vinegar

½ tsp. tarragon, crushed

½ tsp. Dijon mustard

1 cup extra-virgin olive oil

Salt and pepper

Each serving has:
486 calories
15 g carbohydrates
19 g fat
6 g fiber
5 g protein

1. In a large bowl, combine spinach, avocados, olives, onions, cucumber, and oranges. Drizzle with fresh lime juice, paying special attention to coat avocados to prevent browning.

2. In a small saucepan over medium-high heat, bring Balsamic vinegar and tarragon to a boil. Cool for 10 minutes.

3. In a small bowl, combine mustard and vinegar mixture. Stir well.

4. Gradually add oil to vinegar mixture. Whisk until well blended. Season to taste with salt and pepper.

5. Drizzle spinach salad with dressing, and serve.

Spinach Pear Salad

Yield: 8 servings   *Prep time:* 10 minutes
Cook time: None   *Serving size:* 6 ounces

⅓ cup cider vinegar
⅓ cup extra-virgin olive oil
1 TB. Dijon mustard
3 pears, cored and sliced
1 lb. spinach leaves

⅓ cup crumbled bleu cheese
½ cup walnuts, chopped
Salt and pepper

Each serving has:
195 calories
13 g carbohydrates
13 g fat
3 g fiber
6 g protein

1. In a large bowl, whisk cider vinegar, oil, and mustard. Drop pear slices into the bowl, and coat with dressing.

2. Add spinach to the bowl. Toss gently.

3. Sprinkle with bleu cheese and walnuts. Gently mix. Add salt and pepper to taste. Serve.

Chakra Avocado Dip

Yield: 6 servings   *Prep time:* 10 minutes
Cook time: None   *Serving size:* ½ cup

1 large avocado, peeled and mashed

1 TB. lemon juice, freshly squeezed

2 TB. horseradish

2 cloves garlic, minced

2 TB. nonfat yogurt

½ cup nonfat sour cream

Each serving has:
74 calories
6 g carbohydrates
5 g fat
1 g fiber
2 g protein

1. In a medium bowl, combine mashed avocado, lemon juice, horseradish, garlic, yogurt, and sour cream.

2. Stir well. Serve with whole-wheat crackers and vegetable sticks.

Pear Yogurt Bread

Yield: 10 servings   *Prep time:* 10 minutes
Cook time: 50 minutes   *Serving size:* 1 slice

1 cup brown sugar

½ cup non-transfat margarine or light butter

2 large eggs, slightly beaten

1 TB. orange juice

2 medium-ripe pears, shredded

½ cup nonfat yogurt

2 cups whole-wheat flour

1 TB. baking powder

½ tsp. salt

½ cup walnuts, chopped

1 TB. orange zest

Each serving has:
298 calories
39 g carbohydrates
12 g fat
4 g fiber
7 g protein

1. Preheat the oven to 350°F. In a large bowl, cream brown sugar and margarine. Add eggs, and beat well.

2. Gradually stir in orange juice, pears, and yogurt. Set aside.

3. Sift together whole-wheat flour, baking powder, and salt. Stir flour mixture into yogurt mixture.

4. Fold nuts and orange zest into mixture.

5. Pour mixture into a greased, floured loaf pan.

6. Bake for 50 minutes or until a toothpick inserted into center of loaf comes out clean.

Baked Eggs Florentine Casserole

Yield: 8 servings   *Prep time:* 10 minutes
Cook time: 50 minutes   *Serving size:* 1 slice

1 lb. ground turkey

4 large eggs

2¼ cups skim milk

1 can fat-free cream of mushroom soup, condensed

10 oz. frozen spinach, thawed, chopped, and dried

1 cup fresh mushrooms, sliced

1 cup low-fat sharp cheddar cheese, shredded

1 cup low-fat Monterey Jack cheese, shredded

¼ tsp. dry mustard

2½ cups whole-wheat crackers, crumbled

Each serving has:
320 calories
16 g carbohydrates
10 g fat
2 g fiber
26 g protein

1. Heat a skillet coated with nonstick vegetable spray over medium-high heat. Add ground turkey and cook until browned. Drain off fat. Set turkey aside. Preheat oven to 325°F.

2. In a large bowl, whisk eggs and skim milk until well blended. Add soup, spinach, mushrooms, cheeses, and mustard. Mix until well combined.

3. Lightly grease a 9×13-inch baking dish. Spread crackers evenly over the bottom of the dish. Top crackers with browned ground turkey. Pour egg mixture over top turkey.

4. Bake for 50 minutes or until lightly browned on top.

Granny Smith Apple Slaw

Yield: 8 servings   *Prep time:* 15 minutes
Cook time: None   *Serving size:* 1 cup

⅓ cup packed brown sugar

⅓ cup cider vinegar

1½ TB. extra-virgin olive oil

¼ tsp. salt

¼ tsp. black pepper

2 large Granny Smith apples, cored and chopped fine

1 large Red Delicious apple, cored and chopped fine

12 oz. broccoli coleslaw mix

½ cup dried cranberries

2 TB. sunflower seeds, toasted

Each serving has:
97 calories
17 g carbohydrates
4 g fat
1 g fiber
1 g protein

1. To make dressing: whisk together brown sugar, vinegar, oil, salt, and pepper in a medium bowl.

2. To make slaw: combine apples, broccoli slaw, and dried cranberries.

3. Drizzle slaw with dressing. Toss well to combine. Sprinkle with sunflower seeds. Chill for 3 hours and serve.

Celery and Apple Salad

Yield: 6 servings   *Prep time:* 15 minutes
Cook time: None   *Serving size:* 1 cup

1 TB. honey

3 TB. cider vinegar

3 TB. extra-virgin olive oil

Salt and pepper

1 large Red Delicious apple, cored and sliced

2 stalks celery, sliced very thin

1 head iceberg lettuce, washed, dried, and chopped

1 medium red onion, sliced thin

⅓ cup almonds, chopped

1 cup crumbled Gorgonzola cheese

Each serving has:
221 calories
14 g carbohydrates
14 g fat
4 g fiber
7 g protein

1. In a medium bowl, whisk honey, vinegar, oil, salt, and pepper.

2. In a large bowl, toss apple, celery, lettuce, and onion.

3. Drizzle with dressing from the medium bowl. Toss well to combine. Divide into portions.

4. Top with almonds and Gorgonzola cheese. Serve.

Broccoli Soba Noodles

Yield: 6 servings   *Prep time:* 10 minutes
Cook time: 15 minutes   *Serving size:* 1 cup

½ lb. soba noodles

¼ cup low-sodium soy sauce

2 tsp. sugar

2 tsp. dark sesame oil

1 TB. cornstarch

1 TB. rice wine vinegar

1 TB. extra-virgin olive oil

3 cloves garlic, minced

5 cups broccoli, chopped

¼ cup water

½ cup water chestnuts

1 large carrot, peeled and grated

2 tsp. fresh ginger, minced

Each serving has:
204 calories
37 g carbohydrates
4 g fat
3 g fiber
8 g protein

1. Bring 3 quarts salted water to a boil. Add soba noodles to boiling water. Cook for 10 minutes.

2. Drain noodles and rinse with cool water. In a medium bowl, whisk together soy sauce, sugar, sesame oil, cornstarch, and vinegar. Set aside.

3. In a large skillet, add olive oil and garlic to the pan, over medium-high heat. Sauté garlic until lightly browned.

4. Add broccoli, water, water chestnuts, and carrots to the skillet. Cover. Cook for 6 minutes, or until broccoli is tender.

5. Gradually stir in soy sauce mixture. Cook for 5 minutes, or until liquid thickens. Add ginger to skillet.

6. Reduce to low heat. Add soba noodles to the pan. Stir to coat well. Serve.

Exercises to Balance Your Heart Chakra

Let's get started with some personal-growth exercises that will balance your fourth energy center.

Let Go of Your Biggest Heartache

This week, choose to let go of your greatest heartache, and enjoy a vast sense of personal freedom. For this exercise you will need a 3×5-inch index card, a pen, a helium balloon, and approximately 15 inches of string or ribbon. Prior to beginning this exercise, sit quietly and take a few deep, cleansing breaths.

Think about the area of your life that causes you the most heartache or stress. This issue typically triggers emotional eating. This could be the fact that you have gained 30 pounds since your wedding day. Or perhaps you are most troubled by a rocky relationship. Write down your life's greatest heartache and stressor on the index card.

Next, use the ribbon to attach the index card to your helium balloon. Go outside with your balloon. Spend a few minutes thinking about how your greatest stressor has affected your life and your health. Then gently release your balloon into the air, into the wide open space. As your balloon drifts into the sky, imagine that your life's greatest stressor is floating out of your life forever, just like this balloon.

Imagine how wonderful and freeing it feels to have this problem completely removed from your life. Envision that you are giving this problem back to the universe, back to God, or back to any power greater than yourself. Whenever negative feelings resurface, picture this balloon floating away in your mind's eye. This exercise is a great way to let go of anything that seems out of your control. It can be repeated as needed, to release problems and give your heart center a sense of openness and relief.

Recipes for Acts of Love and Kindness

This week, experience true love and compassion by serving others. When you are trying to lose weight and to become a healthier person, it is easy to become self-focused and self-involved. Vow to do something kind for someone else this week and expect nothing in return. It is one of life's greatest paradoxes that by giving things away, you receive the greatest rewards. Open your heart chakra by extending acts of loving kindness to your family, friends, and neighbors. Here are some ideas:

- Bake some goodies and give them away—Whip up a batch of healthy organic cupcakes and take them to your local Ronald McDonald House. Or clear your pantry of excess canned goods and deliver them to your local homeless shelter.

- Give your time away—Instead of watching television, serve someone in need. Volunteer to baby-sit for a single mom, spend an afternoon visiting with an elderly neighbor, or mentor a disadvantaged child in your community.

- Give your talents away. Find a way to offer a needy individual or charitable organization your unique skills. Serve others by doing something that comes easily to you.

- Let go of some loose change. Donate money to your favorite charity or cause. If you are short on cash, find a small way to make a big difference. Writing a ten dollar check to a struggling non-profit is a great way to make a contribution that matters.

- Give away your clutter. The items that are collecting dust in your attic could bring sheer joy to a needy family. Gently used toys, books, clothing, eyeglasses, and cars are all great items to donate.

- Bury the hatchet. Forgiveness is an act of love that will open your heart center and allow compassion to flow back into your life. This week, forgive someone who has wronged you. Just because you decide to forgive someone does not mean that you condone his behavior.

Your Heart's Desire

We all have long-forgotten dreams and things that we long to do, be, or have in life. When these dreams lie dormant, they can clog your heart chakra and cause weight gain. This week is your opportunity to get in touch with your heart's desire.

Sit quietly by yourself in your meditation area. Take a few deep, cleansing breaths. Take some time to figure out what you most want in life. At first, you may think all you want to do is lose 15 pounds and fit into that leopard-print bikini. Imagine that you have achieved your initially desired goal. Now, what do you want next? It may take some time for the answer to surface. The answer may surprise you. Perhaps you have always thought you wanted a million dollars, but what you really long for is a sense of freedom and security. Only you know what you really want and need out of this life.

As you ponder your heart's desire, release others' expectations of you. This is your chance to discover what you really want and need to make you feel happy and fulfilled. Write about your heart's desire in your journal. Try making a collage or picture that illustrates your heart's desire. Draw a picture of yourself happily living out your heart's desire. Hang your picture or collage somewhere you can see it daily. What small step can you take today to attain your heart's desire?

Now that you have an idea of what you want the most, find a way to give exactly what you want to someone else. Ironically, when we give away what we most want to receive, we often find that it comes back to us tenfold. For example, if you most desire a supportive partner who will attend to your emotional needs, make a decision to become that encouraging friend who always lends a listening ear. Or, if you most desire some quality alone time with your partner, offer to baby-sit for the parents of young children so they can enjoy some couple time.

This week, set aside some time to help someone else manifest his heart's desire and expect nothing in return. You will be amazed at how the universe returns the favor directly to your door.

Avalanche of Compliments

As we discussed previously, our heart chakra becomes closed during a stressful, hectic day and we often focus on the negative aspects within ourselves or others. This week, open your heart chakra by catching your family and friends doing positive things. Focus on what they are doing well instead of on what they're doing wrong, or what you think they should be doing. For example, if your partner arrives home late from work and forgets to pick up the dry-cleaning, resist the temptation to comment on his shortcomings. Instead, focus on what he is doing right in the moment. Say, "I am so glad you are home. I really appreciate that you work long hours to help provide for our family."

This technique also works well with strangers. The next time you find yourself interacting with a cranky cashier or postal worker, find something that she is doing skillfully and compliment her.

Be sure to shower yourself with compliments this week. In order for you to truly appreciate others, you must admire yourself first. If you are constantly judging yourself and finding flaws with your body, you will eventually project this behavior outward to others.

In your journal, write at least 10 things that you truly love and admire about yourself. How does it feel to give yourself compliments?

Show Your Love for Yourself and the Environment

According to the Worldwatch Institute, recent research suggests that global warming is occurring right now. Show the earth and yourself why going green is the best way to honor yourself and to lose weight. Following are some suggestions for giving back to the earth by going green:

- Consider walking or riding a bike to work or to run errands— Physical activity will not only help you shed pounds, but it will also cut back on the amount of gas you use and how much you pollute the air. Also look into carpooling options if you live far from work.

- Save energy at home—by setting your thermostat a few degrees lower in the colder months, and a few degrees higher in the warmer months. If you are feeling cold, do some vigorous exercise to warm up your body and protect the environment.

- Take shorter showers and install low-flow showerheads in an effort to conserve water. Use the time you would have spent in the shower to meditate each morning or to add minutes on to your exercise routine.

- Replace your incandescent lightbulbs with long-lasting, lower-energy compact fluorescent bulbs. Investigate the feasibility of wind or solar-energy systems for your home.

- Bring your own reusable tote bags to the grocery store instead of using paper or plastic bags.

- Shop at your local vegetable stand or farmers' market. The produce there is typically organic and tastes better than fruit you buy at the grocery store. The money you spend will go back to your local community and helps save on food related transportation costs.

Establish at least one meat-free day a week. Restricting your meat consumption is one simple way to help you lose weight, save money, and protect the environment. Industrial meat production requires a huge amount of fossil fuel, and releases noxious waste into our air and streams. Buying organic free-range meat is another way to help the environment and one's own health.

Get Physical! Pry Open Your Heart Chakra Through Yoga

Yoga postures are great ways to increase your flexibility, strengthen your muscles, and get the energy flowing to your heart center. This yoga pose is an excellent method to get your heart chakra back in alignment and get physically fit.

The spinal twist, otherwise known as Matsyendrasana in ancient Sanskrit, expands your heart center and massages your chest cavity and thymus gland.

Prior to assuming this posture, take a few deep, cleansing breaths to center yourself and quiet your mind.

Sit on a yoga mat or folded blanket, with your legs stretched out in front of you. Sit up straight with your spine extended and lengthened. Exhale deeply and bend both of your knees. Move your left foot under your right leg. Allow your right knee to point up toward the sky.

On your next inhalation, bring your left arm around the outside of your right knee. With your left hand, grasp your knee or any part of your right foot.

On your next exhalation, press your left arm against your right leg, while twisting your upper body to the right. Be sure to keep your shoulders erect and level. Protect your lower back by engaging your core abdominal muscles.

On your next inhalation, raise your right arm over your head. Slowly exhale and place your palm on the floor next to your buttocks. Inhale deeply.

On your next exhalation, very slowly turn your head to the right. Gently gaze over your right shoulder, if this is comfortable for you.

After you gently release this pose, repeat it on your left side.

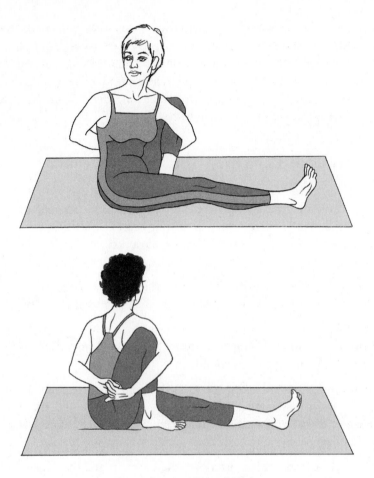

Bound Knee Spinal Twist

A Meditation for Your Heart and Soul

Retreat into your favorite meditation space. Gently close your eyes and become aware of your breathing. Notice any sensations you feel in your body and any thoughts on your mind. Gently let them go.

Breathe in love. Breathe out fear. Continue breathing in love and breathing out fear for 10 breaths.

Imagine a white, healing light in your heart. This light feels so good as it warms every cell in your body. You experience a vast sense of peace like you have never known before.

Continue to breathe in this white, healing light into your heart center.

Now picture a group of your family and friends standing before you. Bring each person forward one at a time. When you exhale, breathe this loving white light from your heart center directly to your loved one's heart center. Spend as much time as you need with each person.

If you choose, you may visualize a person with whom you have a strained or challenging relationship. On your next exhalation, breathe the loving white light from your heart center to this person's heart center. Breathe in forgiveness and breathe out resentment.

At the end of your meditation session, offer gratitude for all of the good people in your life.

5

Your Throat Chakra

About Your Throat Chakra

Your throat chakra is located at the base of the neck near your pharynx, anterior to your windpipe, and it is represented by the color blue. This energy center is physically associated with the thyroid and parathyroid glands. The fifth chakra is associated with sounds, and it involves communication, speech, and self-confidence.

A person with a stagnant throat chakra may have difficulty communicating with others and expressing herself. Signs and symptoms of fifth chakra problems include chronic frustration, social anxiety, dishonesty, and a short attention span. Stuffing your throat full of food, instead of finding your authentic voice is a common occurrence if you are struggling with this energy center. Insidious weight gain often co-exists with a blocked fifth chakra due to a marked inability to communicate and express genuineness.

When the fifth chakra is in balance, you are able to speak your truth and are free to creatively express yourself. A balanced fifth chakra enables you to truly listen to and hear others. A healthy fifth chakra supplies you with ample energy for speaking, singing, thinking, and creative writing.

Stimulate your fifth chakra by wearing blue clothing and blue gemstones, such as lapis, around your neck. After completing this week's exercises, you will be more effectively able to communicate with others and speak your truth.

Let's get started by taking a look at this week's eating plan.

THROAT CHAKRA SEVEN-DAY EATING PLAN

Day One

Breakfast: Blueberry Mango Smoothie
Midmorning Snack: $1/2$ cup blueberries
Lunch: Steak Salad with Bleu Cheese Dressing
Midafternoon Snack: $1/4$ cup raw sunflower seeds
Dinner: Wasabi Mini Crab Cakes
Dessert: Indigo Fruit Salad

Day Two

Breakfast: Berry Crêpes with Honey Orange Sauce
Midmorning Snack: $1/2$ cup nonfat yogurt with fresh blackberries
Lunch: Blue Corn and Gorgonzola Risotto
Midafternoon Snack: 2 cups plain popcorn
Dinner: Spicy Shrimp Tortillas
Dessert: Blueberry and Blackberry Yogurt Parfait

Day Three

Breakfast: Blueberry Wheat Muffin and 1 cup of skim or soy milk
Midmorning Snack: Blueberry Salsa with whole-wheat crackers
Lunch: Blue Fin Tuna Salad
Midafternoon Snack: $1/2$ cup pistachio nuts
Dinner: Shrimp and Crab Penne Drenched in Almost Alfredo Sauce
Dessert: Frozen Grape Delight dipped in Blueberry Salsa

Day Four

Breakfast: Blueberry and Blackberry Yogurt Parfait
Midmorning Snack: 1 large apple
Lunch: Blue Potato Salad
Midafternoon Snack: 10 celery sticks with Blueberry Salsa
Dinner: Wasabi Mini Crab Cakes
Dessert: Elderberries topped with low-fat yogurt and chopped walnuts

Day Five

Breakfast: Nutritious Blueberry Pancakes

Midmorning Snack: $1/2$ cup raisins

Lunch: Indigo Fruit Salad

Midafternoon Snack: 1 hard-boiled egg

Dinner: Grilled Chicken or your choice of fish, topped with Blueberry Salsa (recipe in this chapter)

Dessert: Blueberry Wheat Muffin

Day Six

Breakfast: Berry Crêpes with Honey Orange Sauce

Midmorning Snack: 1 cup nonfat boysenberry yogurt

Lunch: Steak Salad with Bleu Cheese Dressing

Midafternoon Snack: 2 cups plain popcorn

Dinner: Spicy Shrimp Tortillas

Dessert: Blueberries and Cream ($1/2$ cup blueberries topped with $1/4$ cup skim milk)

Day Seven

Breakfast: Blueberry Mango Smoothie

Midmorning Snack: $1/4$ cup whole, raw almonds

Lunch: Indigo Fruit Salad

Midafternoon Snack: $1/2$ cup fat-free cottage cheese

Dinner: Black Bean Burger with Blueberry Salsa

Dessert: Blueberry Wheat Muffin

Foods That Enhance Your Throat Chakra

Fruits and vegetables that contain blue pigments and/or skins are excellent ways to support your fifth energy center and your overall health. In addition, seafood and organic honey are great ways to enhance your throat chakra. Some fruits and vegetables with blue fruits and skins include the following:

Anchovies	Lobster
Blueberries	Mussels
Blackberries	Organic honey
Boysenberries	Salmon
Crabmeat	Sardines
Crayfish	Scallops
Elderberries	Shrimp

Throat Chakra Recipes

Here are this week's gourmet recipes that will enhance your throat chakra.

Spicy Shrimp Tortillas

Yield: 8 servings   *Prep time:* 10 minutes
Cook time: 15 minutes   *Serving size:* 1 taco

4 TB. extra-virgin olive oil

1 clove garlic, minced

2 TB. chili powder

1 lb. large shrimp, peeled
  and deveined

Dash sea salt

Chipotle sauce, to taste

1 red bell pepper, julienned

1 Vidalia onion, julienned

4 TB. lime juice, fresh-
  squeezed

1 cup low-fat cheddar
  cheese, shredded

1 cup romaine lettuce,
  shredded

¼ cup cilantro, minced

8 corn tortillas

Each serving has:
215 calories
11 g carbohydrates
13 g fat
1 g fiber
18 g protein

1. In a large mixing bowl, combine olive oil, garlic, and chili powder. Add shrimp and gently toss to thoroughly coat. Season with sea salt and chipotle sauce to taste. Place the bowl in the refrigerator to marinate for 2 hours.

2. Preheat a griddle over medium-high heat. Place shrimp on skewers. Cook red pepper and onion on the grill for 5 minutes or until tender. Remove peppers and onions from the grill and set aside.

3. Place shrimp skewers on the grill. Cook on each side for about 4 minutes, or until done, depending on thickness of shrimp and the heat of your grill.

4. Remove shrimp from the grill and remove the skewers. Drizzle lime juice over shrimp.

5. Fill tortillas with shrimp, taking care to evenly divide. Top shrimp tortillas with red peppers, onions, cheddar cheese, lettuce, and cilantro.

Blue Corn and Gorgonzola Risotto

Yield: 6 servings   *Prep time:* 10 minutes
Cook time: 25 minutes   *Serving size:* ¾ cup

3 TB. extra-virgin olive oil	½ cup blue cornmeal	*Each serving has:*
1 medium onion, diced fine	¾ cup grated Parmesan cheese	430 calories
5 cups vegetable stock, ready-to-serve	Salt and pepper	55 g carbohydrates
2 cups Arborio rice	1 cup low-fat Gorgonzola cheese	16 g fat
		1 g fiber
		14 g protein

1. Heat olive oil in 4-to-5-quart saucepan over medium heat.

2. Add onion and cook, continuing to stir, until it turns soft and translucent. Turn the heat down if onion starts to brown.

3. Pour vegetable stock into a separate saucepan, set over medium heat, and bring to gentle simmer. Adjust the heat as needed to maintain this simmer the whole time you are preparing risotto.

4. Once onion is soft, add rice and cook over medium heat, stirring constantly, for about 3 minutes.

5. Using a ladle, scoop up about ½ to ¾ cup stock. Pour into the pan with rice, stirring constantly with a spoon.

6. Continue to stir rice constantly, making sure you scrape the bottom of the pan so that it does not stick. If rice reaches a vigorous boil, turn the heat down to medium low.

7. When most of liquid is absorbed into rice, and rice begins to look dry, add another ladle of broth to the pan and stir constantly.

8. Continue to add broth in ½- to ¾-cup batches. Stir rice until you have used most of broth (this probably will take about 20 minutes).

9. Before adding the last amount of stock, stir in blue cornmeal. Then add remaining stock, and stir. Add Parmesan cheese and salt and pepper to taste.

10. When rice is tender, and risotto has a creamy consistency, almost like thick oatmeal, it is done.

11. Spoon risotto onto serving dish and sprinkle with Gorgonzola cheese.

Steak Salad with Bleu Cheese Dressing

Yield: 6 servings   *Prep time:* 10 minutes
Cook time: 10 minutes   *Serving size:* 8 ounces

2 heads romaine lettuce, cut into bite-size pieces

1 large head Belgian endive, sliced thin crosswise

½ red onion, sliced thin into rings

3 cups baby arugula

12 cherry tomatoes, halved

4 oz. Gorgonzola cheese, coarsely crumbled

½ cup red wine vinegar

3 TB. lemon juice

2 tsp. honey

2 tsp. salt

1 tsp. ground black pepper

1 cup olive oil

½ lb. cooked steak, sliced

Each serving has:
510 calories
12 g carbohydrates
30 g fat
5 g fiber
12 g protein

1. In a large bowl, combine romaine lettuce, endive, red onion, arugula, cherry tomatoes, and half cheese.

2. Mix vinegar, lemon juice, honey, salt, and pepper in a blender. With the machine running, gradually blend in oil. Toss salad with enough vinaigrette to coat.

3. Season salad with salt and pepper, to taste. Arrange salad on a platter.

4. Cut steaks crosswise into thin slices. Arrange steak slices atop salad and sprinkle with remaining cheese.

5. Drizzle more vinaigrette over steak slices and serve family-style.

Shrimp and Crab Penne Drenched in Almost Alfredo Sauce

Yield: 6 servings   *Prep time:* 10 minutes
Cook time: 10 minutes   *Serving size:* 1 cup

¾ cup nonfat Parmesan cheese, grated

½ cup low-fat ricotta cheese

½ cup evaporated skim milk

⅛ tsp. white pepper, ground

Dash ground nutmeg

2⅔ cups skim milk

½ lb. lump crabmeat, cooked

⅓ lb. shrimp, cooked, peeled, and chopped

4 cups whole-wheat penne pasta

Each serving has:
421 calories
62 g carbohydrates
6 g fat
6 g fiber
35 g protein

1. In a medium bowl, combine Parmesan cheese, ricotta cheese, evaporated milk, pepper, and nutmeg. Mix well and set aside.

2. In a saucepan over medium heat, bring skim milk to boil, stirring frequently to avoid scalding. Add contents of the medium bowl to the saucepan. Stir for 2 minutes until sauce thickens.

3. Gently stir in cooked crab, cooked shrimp, and cooked whole-wheat penne pasta. Toss well to coat shellfish and pasta. Serve.

Berry Crêpes with Honey Orange Sauce

Yield: 4 servings   *Prep time:* 10 minutes
Cook time: None   *Serving size:* 2 crêpes

1 cup fresh blueberries

1 cup sliced strawberries

1 TB. sugar

9 oz. low-fat cream cheese,
softened

¼ cup organic honey

¾ cup orange juice

8 crêpes (6½ inches)

Each serving has:
278 calories
38 g carbohydrates
10 g fat
2 g fiber
8 g protein

1. Combine blueberries, strawberries, and sugar in a small bowl. Set aside.

2. To prepare sauce, beat cream cheese and honey until well blended. Slowly beat in orange juice.

3. Spoon ¹/₂ cup of berry filling in center of 1 crêpe. Spoon 1 tablespoon sauce over berries. Roll up. Place on a serving plate. Repeat with remaining crêpes.

4. Pour remaining sauce over crêpes.

Blue Fin Tuna Salad

Yield: 2 servings   *Prep time:* 10 minutes
Cook time: None   *Serving size:* 6 ounces

10 oz. blue fin tuna, cooked, and cooled, or canned tuna

6 TB. red onion, diced fine

6 TB. celery, diced fine

2 TB. pickle, diced fine

1 TB. brown mustard

6 TB. nonfat mayonnaise

1 tsp. lemon juice

1 TB. tarragon

Salt and pepper

2 cups chopped lettuce leaves

Each serving has:
281 calories
38 g carbohydrates
8 g fat
2 g fiber
36 g protein

1. Place tuna in a large bowl and lightly break apart tuna. Mix with onions, celery, and pickles. Set aside.

2. In a medium bowl, mix mustard, mayonnaise, lemon juice, tarragon, salt, and pepper.

3. Add tuna mix to dressing. Combine until tuna is coated evenly.

4. Serve over bed of lettuce.

Blue Potato Salad

Yield: 6 servings   *Prep time:* 10 minutes
Cook time: 18 minutes   *Serving size:* 8 ounces

1 cup edamame

4 red potatoes, peeled

4 blue potatoes, peeled

1 TB. mustard seeds

Black pepper, to taste

1 cup low-fat sour cream

½ cup low-fat mayonnaise

1 cup low-fat bleu cheese

2 green onions, chopped

1 stalk celery, chopped

1 TB. cider vinegar

½ cup fresh dill, chopped

Each serving has:
152 calories
16 g carbohydrates
8 g fat
1 g fiber
4 g protein

1. Fill a salted stockpot with 3 quarts salted water. Boil edamame for 10 minutes. Drain, and allow to cool.

2. In a separate stockpot, boil red and blue potatoes in 5 quarts water for 15 minutes. Drain. Allow potatoes to cool and dice into ¹/₂-inch pieces.

3. In a large bowl, combine mustard seed, black pepper, sour cream, and mayonnaise. Mix well.

4. Add bleu cheese, potatoes, green onions, edamame, celery, cider vinegar, and dill. Combine.

5. Cover and place the bowl in the refrigerator overnight to chill. Serve.

Wasabi Mini Crab Cakes

Yield: 6 servings   *Prep time:* 10 minutes
Cook time: 10 minutes   *Serving size:* 2 crab cakes

1 pint lump crabmeat

⅓ cup green bell pepper, diced fine

⅓ cup red bell pepper, diced fine

⅓ cup green onion, chopped fine

1 cup whole kernel corn, frozen (or use fresh)

⅓ cup light mayonnaise

¾ cup whole-wheat breadcrumbs

1 egg, beaten

½ cup cornmeal

¼ cup olive oil

3 TB. wasabi powder

¼ cup low-fat mayonnaise

¼ cup low-fat sour cream

⅓ cup Dijon mustard

¼ cup scallions, chopped fine

Each serving has:
271 calories
32 g carbohydrates
9 g fat
4 g fiber
14 g protein

1. In a large bowl, combine crabmeat, green pepper, red pepper, green onion, corn, mayonnaise, breadcrumbs, and egg.

2. Shape crabmeat into 12 equal-size small cakes.

3. Place cornmeal in a shallow dish. Dredge each crab cake in cornmeal to coat. Coat both sides.

4. In a large skillet over medium-low heat, add olive oil.

5. Pan fry crab cakes until golden brown, approximately 4 minutes on each side.

6. To make sauce, combine wasabi, mayonnaise, sour cream, and mustard. Gradually blend in scallions. Garnish crab cakes with sauce.

Nutritious Blueberry Pancakes

Yield: 2 servings   *Prep time:* 10 minutes
Cook time: 6 minutes   *Serving size:* 2 small pancakes

½ pint nonfat yogurt

¼ cup whole-wheat flour

1 large egg, beaten

½ tsp. baking soda

½ cup blueberries

½ cup polenta

1 TB. extra-virgin olive oil

4 TB. nonfat cream
   cheese, softened

Each serving has:

480 calories

79 g carbohydrates

10 g fat

10 g fiber

18 g protein

1. In a large bowl, combine yogurt, whole-wheat flour, egg, baking soda, blueberries, and polenta.

2. In a large skillet or griddle over medium-high heat, add olive oil.

3. Drop 3 tablespoons blueberry batter into the pan. Cook for 2 minutes on each side, until lightly golden.

4. Top pancake with dollop of fat-free cream cheese. Serve while warm.

Blueberry Mango Smoothie

Yield: 2 servings   *Prep time:* 10 minutes
Cook time: None   *Serving size:* 1½ cups

1 large mango, peeled and chopped

I large banana, peeled and sliced

1 cup blueberries

1 TB. honey

1 TB. flaxseed oil

1 cup nonfat plain yogurt

½ cup skim milk

½ cup ice cubes

Each serving has:
312 calories
61 g carbohydrates
1 g fat
4 g fiber
19 g protein

1. Place mango, banana, blueberries, honey, flaxseed oil, yogurt, skim milk, and ice cubes in a blender.

2. Purée on high speed until thoroughly blended. Serve immediately.

Blueberry Wheat Muffins

Yield: 12 servings   *Prep time:* 10 minutes
Cook time: 30 minutes   *Serving size:* 1 muffin

1 large egg	2 tsp. baking powder	*Each serving has:*
¼ cup vegetable oil	2 tsp. flaxseed oil	175 calories
½ cup skim milk	½ tsp. salt	23 g carbohydrates
1½ cups whole-wheat flour	½ cup walnuts, chopped	8 g fat
½ cup sugar	1 cup fresh blueberries	2 g fiber
		4 g protein

1. Preheat the oven to 400°F. Grease a standard muffin tin, or line muffin tins with paper baking cups.

2. In a large bowl, beat egg. Gradually stir in oil and milk.

3. Gradually add whole-wheat flour, sugar, baking powder, flaxseed oil, salt, walnuts, and blueberries.

4. Stir until flour is moistened. Batter will be lumpy.

5. Pour batter into the muffin tins. Fill the muffin cups ²/₃ full.

6. Bake for 20 to 22 minutes until golden brown, and a knife inserted into the center of muffin comes out clean.

7. Remove from the pan and cool for 15 minutes. Serve.

Blueberry and Blackberry Yogurt Parfait

Yield: 1 serving   *Prep time:* 10 minutes
Cook time: None   *Serving size:* 1 tall parfait glass

¼ cup almonds, chopped
⅓ cup blueberries
⅓ cup blackberries

1 large banana, sliced
8 oz. nonfat vanilla yogurt

Each serving has:
567 calories
87 g carbohydrates
17 g fat
11 g fiber
21 g protein

1. Place ¹/₃ almonds in a tall parfait glass. Set aside. In a medium bowl, gently stir blueberries, blackberries, and bananas into yogurt.

2. Place ¹/₃ yogurt and fruit mixture on top chopped almonds. Top with almonds.

3. Repeat layers. Top with remaining almonds. Serve immediately.

Indigo Fruit Salad

Yield: 6 servings   *Prep time:* 15 minutes
Cook time: None; refrigerate 3 hours   *Serving size:* 1 cup

1 pint strawberries, halved

1 large mango, peeled and diced

1 large plum, diced

1 large peach, pitted and chopped

1 cup blackberries

1 cup blueberries

¼ cup organic honey

2 TB. lemon juice, fresh-squeezed

1 TB. lemon zest

1 large banana, sliced

Each serving has:
139 calories
36 g carbohydrates
1 g fat
5 g fiber
1 g protein

1. In a large bowl, combine strawberries, mango, plum, peach, blackberries, and blueberries. Add honey, lemon juice, and lemon zest. Toss well.

2. Cover and chill for at least 3 hours. Add sliced bananas to salad just prior to serving.

Blueberry Salsa

Yield: 6 servings   *Prep time:* 15 minutes
Cook time: None; refrigerate overnight   *Serving size:* ¼ cup

2 cups blueberries, coarsely chopped	3 TB. cilantro, chopped fine
½ cup whole-kernel corn, frozen	¼ cup lime juice, fresh-squeezed
½ medium Vidalia onion, chopped fine	1 tsp. kosher salt
1 small jalapeño, seeded and chopped	Celery sticks
	Carrot sticks
1 small red bell pepper, seeded and chopped	Red pepper sticks

Each serving has:
56 calories
14 g carbohydrates
Trace fat
2 g fiber
1 g protein

1. In a large bowl, combine blueberries, corn, onion, jalapeño, red pepper, cilantro, lime juice, and salt. Stir well.

2. Refrigerate overnight to allow flavors to blend together. Serve with celery sticks, carrot sticks, and red pepper strips.

Black Bean Burgers with Blueberry Salsa

Yield: 4 servings   *Prep time:* 25 minutes
Cook time: 15 minutes   *Serving size:* 1 burger

½ cup bulgur, medium-grind

¼ tsp. sea salt

1 cup boiling water

1 (15 oz.) can black beans, rinsed and drained

¼ cup whole-wheat bread-crumbs

4 green onions, chopped fine

1 large egg

1 sweet potato, shredded

1 large carrot, grated

¼ tsp. cayenne pepper

2 TB. tahini

Salt and pepper

2 TB. olive oil

½ cup Blueberry Salsa (recipe in this chapter)

4 whole-wheat English muffins, halved and toasted

Each serving has:
660 calories
117 g carbohydrates
9 g fat
25 g fiber
34 g protein

1. In a large bowl, mix bulgur with sea salt and 1 cup of boiling water. Cover the bowl. Allow the bowl to stand for 30 minutes so bulgur can become tender. Drain bulgur in sieve.

2. In a medium bowl, mash black beans with a fork. Add breadcrumbs, green onions, egg, sweet potato, carrot, cayenne pepper, tahini, and bulgur.

3. Season with salt and pepper to taste. Shape mixture into 4 (1-inch-thick) patties.

4. Heat olive oil over medium-high heat in a large skillet. Cook burger patties until brown and firm, approximately 6 minutes on each side.

5. Top each burger with 2 tablespoons of Blueberry Salsa and serve on toasted English muffin.

Exercises to Balance Your Throat Chakra

Let's get started with some personal-growth exercises that will balance your fifth energy center.

Listen and Pay Attention with Your Whole Body

We all are born with an internal radar system that alerts us to danger and lets us know when we need to be on guard. For example, when we encounter a dangerous situation or person, oftentimes our arm hair will stand on end and our heart rate will increase before we actually see the threat with our eyes. Like an animal who moves to higher ground prior to a flood, we posses an internal radar that protects us from harm.

We constantly take in information from our environment on many different levels. Much of this data is nonverbal, intuitive, and difficult to explain. Observe how a young child reacts to a phony adult and you will see this theory in action. Over time, our minds and our bodies can become disconnected, and this inner knowing can become lessened. Instead of paying attention to our body's intrinsic warning system, we learn to rely on our thinking.

This week, reconnect to your animal instincts and internal sense of knowing. When someone is talking to you, listen to him with your whole body, not simply with your ears and your brain.

Start by paying attention to your breathing when you are in a dialogue with another person. Does your breath quicken or become shallow when certain people speak with you? Do you feel safe and supported in the presence of others? What signals is your body sending to you? When you speak, do you feel any tightness in your throat? Or does it feel relaxed and supple? What is your body trying to tell you? In your journal, imagine that you are your throat. What is your throat trying to tell you? If your whole body could talk, what would it say?

Listen to your body before you place any food in your mouth. For example, before placing that piece of chocolate cake in your mouth, ask your body if it truly wants to receive this piece of junk food. Sit quietly for at least five minutes and listen for your body's answer. By this time, your craving should pass, and you will have enough time to tune into your body's true desire.

Silence Is Golden

Most of us live in a noisy world. From the moment we arise in the morning, our ears are bombarded with constant clamoring. The television blares in the background, sirens wail on the street, and our neighbor's stereo system blasts. We sit at work in a sea of cubicles among nonstop chatter and chaos.

In the midst of all this upheaval, it is easy to stop listening to our own inner voice. Many of us turn to food to cope with the turmoil.

This week, retreat from the noisy world for 24 consecutive hours. Vow to spend one full day in silence. During this time, you should not speak with anyone, nor should anyone speak with you, unless of course, there is an absolute emergency.

Unplug your television, telephone, and computer. Resist the temptation to check your e-mail or the football score. Use this time to practice your meditation skills. Focus on just being, instead of on doing or accomplishing anything. Experiment with various journaling exercises in this book in an effort to get to know yourself better. Connect with your personal sense of inner peace through the silence.

The authors of *The Inner Peace Diet* hold several silent retreat weekends each year. During these retreats, participants enjoy silence in a beautiful, natural setting and are served delicious whole foods. Talking and open dialogue is encouraged at hour-long workshops, and individual sessions are held each evening. The retreats are a life-transforming experience that teach participants how to access inner peace through silence. For more information on our silent-retreat weekends, please visit www.innerpeacediet.com. Alternatively, there are other options for silent retreats all around the world. Find the journey into silence that suits you best.

Get Physical! Open Up Your Throat Chakra Through Yoga

Practicing yoga postures that focus on stimulating and expanding your throat chakra is a great way to activate weight loss and bliss. The Half Fish pose, known as Matsyasana in Sanskrit, is one surefire way to get energy flowing to your fifth energy center.

To assume the Half Fish pose, lie on your back and extend your legs out in front of you. Take a few minutes to breathe deeply and quiet your mind. Place your hands close together, underneath your buttocks. Make sure that your palms are facing down and your fingers are free of tension. Adjust your legs so that they are close together. Release all of the stress from your legs, and allow your whole body to be at peace.

When you are ready, inhale as you gently lift the weight of your whole body onto your elbows. Allow your neck to safely tilt backward so that the back of your head rests on the floor. Arch your back, and let your legs relax on the floor. Shift all of your weight onto your elbows. Firmly press your buttocks onto the floor.

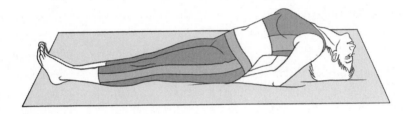

Half Fish Pose

Attempt to hold this pose for five whole breaths. Honor your own body first, and release the pose whenever it feels right for you. Release this position by pressing your elbows into the floor. Carefully lift your head and very slowly lower your entire body back to the ground, one vertebrae at a time.

If you have a history of neck problems, please consult your doctor prior to doing this pose.

Shrug Your Throat Chakra Back into Alignment

The Shoulder Shrug Pose, known as Amshavrttanasana in Sanskrit, improves flexibility in the upper-back shoulders and arms as it releases stagnant energy in your fifth chakra.

To assume this yoga pose, sit in any position that feels comfortable to you. You may choose to sit with your legs crossed at the ankles, or you may sit on a chair. Alternatively, you may do this pose while in Mountain Pose, discussed in Chapter 1. Take a few minutes to scan your body for tension and release any tightness in your muscles. Clear your mind of any thoughts, and draw in a few deep, cleansing breaths.

On your next inhalation, gently raise your shoulders up toward the sky until your body tells you to release them.

On your next exhalation, gradually lower your shoulders. Repeat this gentle shrugging and releasing movement in sync with your breath for three minutes.

Notice the immediate difference you feel in your body. Feel how loose and relaxed the muscles in your upper body are in this moment.

Just Press Record

This week, discover the power of your speaking voice and learn to vocalize your truth. Record your speaking voice while you are having a natural conversation or in a dialogue with another person. If you capture someone else's voice on your recording, please be sure to have his permission first.

Listen to this recording when you are alone and have time for contemplation. Take out your journal and write about your experience of your own voice. Does the sound of your voice make you cringe? Many times when clients hear their own voice, they incredulously exclaim, "Is that really me?" or, "I don't sound like *that*!" Do you find your inflection to be pleasant and calming? Does your tone sound forced or contrived? Do you feel that your voice reflects your authentic self? Do you hear any un-expressed anger or sadness in your voice? Do you whisper or mumble instead of using your throat to project your power and wisdom? Do you sound subservient, or do you attempt to dominate every conversation? Is your voice raspy, or is it smooth?

List as many qualities of your voice as you can. Focus on how the sound of your voice makes you feel. When we are overweight, our self-concept takes a beating. We develop a poor body image, and feelings of unworthiness and self-doubt emerge. Many times we deny our own painful feelings and pretend as if nothing is wrong. One way to get out of denial and connect with your truth is to record yourself in conversation. It is easy to discern how you actually feel about yourself when you listen to the sound of your own voice.

This week, experiment with your voice and tone. Imagine that you were healthy, peaceful, and at your goal weight. How would you speak if you were the person you always wanted to be? Would your voice reflect a more confident and authoritative spirit? Pick a person who you truly admire. Attempt to emulate her speaking voice, while still expressing your own unique style and truth. Record your newfound voice. Do you hear the difference? Does your new manner of speaking more accurately express your authentic self?

Scream Your Way to a Healthy Body

Releasing and discharging negative emotion is a necessary part of life. Many people are taught from an early age that it is unacceptable to express anger or sadness, and they subsequently learn to deny their feelings. Some people use food in an effort to numb their feelings, while others simply shut down or space out in an effort to find relief. Repressed anger and pent-up frustration are stored deep within our bodies and in our chakra systems. These feelings often lie just below the surface of our awareness, and can sabotage our weight-loss goals if they are not addressed. Unfortunately, emotions are not an optional part of life. If we do not manage our emotions effectively, they soon will begin to manage us. Emotions stored within our bodies tend to get stuck at our throat chakra. Because we are socially conditioned to say nice things and not tell others how we really feel, this energy gets trapped right near our larynx.

This week, release these toxic emotions and get the energy flowing to your fifth chakra center. Assume a comfortable seated position in a private place. It is important that you find a place where you will not be disturbed or feel embarrassed to shout or scream. It is also important to do this exercise in a place where you will not disturb others, as this exercise could potentially scare others, especially children. You may choose to do this exercise in a secluded area out in nature, or alone in your home.

Gently close your eyes and focus on your breathing. Think of how carrying excess weight makes you feel. Be gentle with yourself. Allow all of your feelings to surface. Welcome each feeling as it arises. Do not try to resist it or push it away. Know that it is more painful to avoid emotions than it is to experience them fully and let them go. Slowly open your mouth and release any negative emotions you feel.

Allow whatever sound is in your throat to be released into the universe. This sound may resemble a whisper, or perhaps it is more like a scream. Attempt to discharge your repressed negative feelings through your voice. You may find that screaming, crying, shouting, laughing, or yodeling are effective ways to discharge these feelings. Each person's process is different. When you feel as if you have finished, record your experiences with this exercise in your journal.

Get Some Support

Human beings are social creatures. We are not designed to live in isolation. Due to the changing nature of our global economy, a sense of community often is missing from our lives. People often eat alone, shop alone, and live great distances from their families of origin and childhood friends. This can leave people feeling disconnected, unsupported, and generally out of sorts.

We need encouragement from others most when we are undergoing a life change. Losing weight and attempting to gain a more peaceful life are major life transitions. People who have shared experiences similar to ours can offer us a great deal of support and comfort. This week, seek to expand your social support network. Attend a support-group meeting in your town. Join an online message board or list-serv for people trying to lose weight.

Practice asking others for help when you need a hand. Although it may not be easy to ask others for assistance, it certainly does feel good to be connected to people who care about you. Join a book club or take a painting class at the nearest community college. Find a new way to connect and seek support from others.

Fight Food Cravings Through Music

On your journey to weight loss and inner bliss, you likely will experience some challenging days. You may experience intense food cravings or undergo mood changes as you adapt to your new, healthy lifestyle. One surefire way to elevate your mood and stop a food craving dead in its tracks is through music. Music is a powerful medium that has the ability to lift your mood instantly and shift your thoughts.

In your journal, write down your top-10 favorite songs of all time. Think back to songs you adored during your childhood and adolescence. Write about the positive emotions you feel when you hear these particular tunes. Whenever you experience a negative emotion or food craving, play one of your favorite songs. Listen to the sound with your whole body. Give yourself permission to dance and sing along. If you are feeling adventurous, this is a great time to learn how to play a musical instrument or pick up that instrument you abandoned long ago.

Sound Meditation

The use of sound during meditation is an ancient practice that cultures have used for centuries. Sound frequency is made up of vibrations that travel through the air. Our chakras can be altered and balanced by these sound meditations. By chanting certain words or phrases, we are able to raise our body's vibrational rate and improve our physical and emotional health. Although this may sound like science fiction, it is a real fact that is steadily gaining recognition.

Our body's vibrations can be measured by special machines that measure and calibrate our electromagnetic field. By increasing our vibration, we gain access to a vast sense of health and inner peace. When we live in a higher vibrational frequency, we lose weight more readily and are more able to fend off disease and stress. In addition, we can create the lives we truly want for ourselves while serving those in need.

Sound meditation balances all of the chakras and provides an instant feeling of tranquility. To begin your personal sound meditation, assume a seated posture that is comfortable for you. Take care to sit with your spine extended and erect. Allow yourself to completely relax in this moment. Take a few deep, cleansing breaths. Gently close your eyes and focus your attention on your throat.

Allow the backs of your hands to softly rest on your knees. Hold your hands with your palms facing up toward the sky. Touch your index fingers to your thumbs. This hand position will help you receive positive energy and increase your vibrational rate.

In your mind's eye picture a blank television screen. Gently let go of any thoughts or worries. Focus on breathing in and breathing out.

Silently or out loud, begin chanting the following words:

- Sa (This word means infinity.)
- Ta (This word means life.)
- Om (This word means the union of mind, body, and soul.)

Repeat each word five times. As you say the word, focus on feeling your energy move from your root chakra up to your throat chakra. Allow this energy to flow up from your throat to the crown of your head. At the end of this meditation, sit quietly for a few minutes and notice how peaceful you are in the moment.

6

Your Third-Eye Chakra

The sixth chakra is called the third-eye chakra, and is associated with both intuitive and physical sight and vision. Through this chakra, we receive inner guidance and tune into our inherent wisdom. The sixth chakra is associated with the color indigo and/or purple and is enhanced by wearing indigo and purple clothing and gemstones.

When the third-eye chakra is unbalanced, a person may have difficulty with memory, unexplained phobias, or decision-making. Signs and symptoms of sixth chakra problems include chronic headaches, vision problems, and obsessive or compulsive thinking.

Emotional eating and weight gain cloud a person's third-eye center and vision. When we are overweight, it is easy to stop seeing ourselves as we truly are. Due to our bruised self-esteem, we avoid looking in the mirror and are in denial about how we actually look and feel.

Excess weight also can cause us to lose our natural sense of intuition. Because we live in a state of avoidance and denial, we fail to see the little guideposts that lead us to our destiny. After implementing the eating plans and exercises in this chapter, you will develop an ability to trust in your inner wisdom and intuitive powers.

Let's get started by taking a look at this week's eating plan.

THIRD-EYE CHAKRA SEVEN-DAY EATING PLAN

Day One

Breakfast: Purple Third-Eye Smoothie
Midmorning Snack: ¼ cup raisins
Lunch: Gazpacho Salad
Midafternoon Snack: 1 cup nonfat cottage cheese
Dinner: Pesto Chicken Salad with Red Grapes
Dessert: Cherry Clafoutis

Day Two

Breakfast: Cheesy Chakra Eggplant Omelet
Midmorning Snack: 1 large bunch red grapes
Lunch: Vivacious Violet Hummus with Veggies
Midafternoon Snack: 1 cup plain popcorn
Dinner: Blackened Cajun Chicken with Purple Smashed Potatoes
Dessert: Third-Eye Purple Sorbet

Day Three

Breakfast: Flaxseed Raisin Bread and ½ cup skim milk or soy milk
Midmorning Snack: ½ cup nonfat yogurt and ½ cup dried pitted plums
Lunch: Pesto Chicken Salad with Red Grapes
Midafternoon Snack: 1 apple
Dinner: Eggplant Caponata
Dessert: Walnut Fig Bar

Day Four

Breakfast: Purple Third-Eye Smoothie
Midmorning Snack: ¼ cup almonds
Lunch: Spiced Red Cabbage, Apple, and Chestnut Salad
Midafternoon Snack: 1 plum
Dinner: Visionary Eggplant Parmesan
Dessert: Baked Plum and Peach Delight

Day Five

Breakfast: Flaxseed Raisin Bread and $1/2$ cup skim milk or soy milk

Midmorning Snack: 1 slice low-fat cheese

Lunch: Gazpacho Salad

Midafternoon Snack: $1/4$ cup raisins

Dinner: Eggplant Mozzarella Wraps

Dessert: Cherry Clafoutis

Day Six

Breakfast: Plum Bran Muffin and $1/2$ cup skim milk or soy milk

Midmorning Snack: 1 cup nonfat cottage cheese

Lunch: Pesto Chicken Salad with Red Grapes

Midafternoon Snack: Walnut Fig Bar

Dinner: Eggplant Caponata

Dessert: Third-Eye Purple Sorbet

Day Seven

Breakfast: Cheesy Chakra Eggplant Omelet

Midmorning Snack: 1 slice cantaloupe sprinkled with raisins

Lunch: Red Cabbage and Red Grape Basil Slaw

Midafternoon Snack: Walnut Fig Bar

Dinner: Eggplant Mozzarella Wraps

Dessert: Baked Plum and Peach Delight

Foods That Enhance Your Third-Eye Chakra

Fruits and vegetables that contain purple or indigo pigments and/or skins are excellent ways to support your sixth energy center and your overall health.

Some fruits and vegetables with purple and indigo pigments and skins include the following:

- Black currants
- Dried plums
- Eggplant
- Plums
- Purple figs
- Purple peppers
- Raisins
- Red cabbage
- Red grapes

Third-Eye Chakra Recipes

Here are this week's gourmet recipes that will enhance your third-eye chakra.

Visionary Eggplant Parmesan

Yield: 6 servings   *Prep time:* 2 hours
Cook time: 35 minutes   *Serving size:* 1 cup

1 large eggplant, sliced into ½-inch-thick rounds

1 TB. salt

6 TB. extra-virgin olive oil

1 red onion, sliced paper-thin

2 roasted red peppers, cut into thin strips

6 TB. Romano cheese, grated

2 TB. Italian seasoning

1 pint low-sodium marinara sauce

¼ lb. provolone cheese, sliced ¼-inch thick

1 TB. fresh parsley, minced

Each serving has:
357 calories
22 g carbohydrates
18 g fat
7 g fiber
13 g protein

1. Place eggplant rounds on baking sheets lined with paper towels. Sprinkle rounds with salt. Let stand for 2 hours to draw out bitterness. Pat dry.

2. Preheat the oven to 350°F.

3. Heat a large skillet over medium-high heat. Add olive oil. Cook eggplant slices until lightly browned on each side. Drain eggplant on paper towels.

4. Place eggplant in a greased 11×13-inch baking dish. Layer eggplant with onion, roasted red pepper strips, Romano cheese, Italian seasoning, and marinara sauce. Repeat layers one time. Top with provolone slices and parsley.

5. Bake for 35 minutes or until lightly browned.

Plum Bran Muffins

Yield: 12 servings   *Prep time:* 15 minutes
Cook time: 18 minutes   *Serving size:* 1 muffin

1¼ cups whole-wheat flour
½ cup soy flour
1 cup bran-flakes cereal
½ cup dark brown sugar
1 tsp. baking powder
1 tsp. baking soda
1 tsp. ground cinnamon
⅛ tsp. ground cloves

2 large eggs, slightly beaten
½ cup soy milk
2 TB. flaxseed oil
¼ cup canola oil
½ cup walnuts
½ cup plums, chopped

Each serving has:
184 calories
21 g carbohydrates
9 g fat
4 g fiber
13 g protein

1. Preheat the oven to 400°F. Spray a muffin pan with nonstick vegetable oil cooking spray.

2. In a large bowl, combine whole-wheat flour, soy flour, bran flakes, brown sugar, baking powder, baking soda, cinnamon, and cloves.

3. In a separate bowl, mix eggs, soy milk, flaxseed oil, and canola oil.

4. Add egg mixture to flour mixture. Stir until blended.

5. Fold in walnuts and plums.

6. Fill the muffin pan ⅔ full.

7. Bake for 16 to 18 minutes, or until a toothpick inserted into center of muffin comes out clean.

Blackened Cajun Chicken

Yield: 6 servings   *Prep time:* 10 minutes
Cook time: 30 minutes   *Serving size:* ¼ pound

1 tsp. paprika
½ tsp. ground cumin
½ tsp. salt
½ tsp. dried thyme
½ tsp. white pepper

¼ tsp. onion powder
¼ tsp. Cajun seasoning
3 TB. safflower oil
1½ lb. chicken breast,
boned and skinned

Each serving has:
199 calories
1 g carbohydrates
13 g fat
Trace fiber
19 g protein

1. Preheat the oven to 350°F.

2. In a medium bowl, combine paprika, ground cumin, salt, thyme, white pepper, onion powder, and Cajun seasoning. Rub one side chicken breast with seasoning mixture.

3. Heat oil in a cast-iron skillet for 5 minutes.

4. Place chicken in a hot pan with the seasoned side face down. Cook for 1 minute. Flip chicken over, and cook for 1 minute on other side.

5. Bake chicken in an ovenproof pan for 10 minutes in the oven. Chicken is done when reaches internal temperature of 165°F. Serve.

Purple Smashed Potatoes

Yield: 6 servings   *Prep time:* 10 minutes
Cook time: 15 minutes   *Serving size:* 1 cup

1½ lb. purple potatoes,
   peeled and quartered

¼ tsp. dried thyme

3 TB. horseradish

½ tsp. salt

⅛ tsp. fresh ground
   pepper

3 TB. skim milk

Each serving has:
144 calories
33 g carbohydrates
Trace fat
3 g fiber
4 g protein

1. Cook potatoes uncovered in a 4-quart stockpot boiling water for 15 minutes or until tender. Drain.

2. In a large stockpot, mash purple potatoes with a potato masher or fork.

3. Add thyme, horseradish, salt, and pepper. Gradually beat in skim milk. Add more milk for lighter, fluffier potatoes. Serve.

Walnut Fig Bars

Yield: 20 servings   *Prep time:* 10 minutes; plus 3 hours to chill dough
Cook time: 35 minutes   *Serving size:* 1 bar

3 cups whole-wheat flour	1 ½ cups dark brown sugar	**Each serving has:**
1 tsp. baking powder	2 large eggs	303 calories
½ tsp. baking soda	2 tsp. vanilla	46 g carbohydrates
1 tsp. cinnamon	1 cup walnuts, chopped	12 g fat
½ tsp. salt	1 lb. dried figs	6 g fiber
¼ cup vegetable shortening	1 TB. flaxseed oil	5 g protein
½ cup light butter, softened	¾ cup orange juice	
¼ cup wheat germ	¼ cup water	

1. Sift together flour, baking powder, baking soda, cinnamon, and salt.

2. In a medium bowl, beat shortening, butter, wheat germ, and 1 cup brown sugar with a mixer on high speed until thoroughly blended.

3. Gradually add in eggs and vanilla. Add flour mixture, and beat until moistened. Gradually stir in walnuts.

4. Flatten dough. Chill dough in the refrigerator for 3 hours.

5. Meanwhile, in a large saucepan over medium-high heat, combine figs, $^1/_2$ cup brown sugar, flaxseed oil, orange juice, and water. Stir mixture constantly for 10 minutes, or until mixture comes to a boil and thickens. Remove from heat. Cool fig filling.

6. Preheat the oven to 350°F. Remove dough from the refrigerator. Divide dough into 2 halves.

7. On a lightly floured surface, roll out $^1/_2$ dough into a 13×9-inch rectangle with a floured rolling pin.

8. Press other $^1/_2$ dough into bottom of a greased 13×9-inch baking pan.

9. Spread fig and orange juice mixture on dough in the baking pan.

10. Carefully place rolled dough rectangle over fig filling.

11. Bake for 35 minutes or until dough is golden brown.

Eggplant Caponata

Yield: 6 servings   *Prep time:* 15 minutes
Cook time: 25 minutes   *Serving size:* 1 cup

2 TB. extra-virgin olive oil

2 medium red onions, chopped

4 cloves garlic, minced

1 stalk celery, chopped

2 large red bell peppers, chopped

1 cup shiitake mushrooms, sliced

1 large eggplant, cubed

3 cups chopped tomatoes

2 TB. capers, drained

¼ cup green olives, pitted and sliced

¼ cup Balsamic vinegar

1 TB. sugar

Salt and pepper

Each serving has:
247 calories
50 g carbohydrates
2 g fat
9 g fiber
6 g protein

1. In a large saucepan, heat 1 tablespoon olive oil over medium-high heat. Sauté onions and garlic until lightly browned.

2. Add celery, red peppers, and mushrooms. Cook vegetables until crispy and tender. Remove from the pan and set aside.

3. Add additional tablespoon olive oil to the saucepan. Brown eggplant for 5 minutes on each side or until tender.

4. Return onions, garlic, red peppers, and mushrooms to the pan.

5. Add tomatoes, capers, olives, vinegar, and sugar to the pan. Season with salt and pepper.

6. Allow to simmer for 15 minutes or until sauce has thickened.

Red Cabbage and Red Grape Basil Slaw

Yield: 10 servings   *Prep time:* 20 minutes
Cook time: None; refrigerate for 1 hour   *Serving size:* 1 cup

½ bunch red seedless
   grapes, washed

½ cup apple cider vinegar

1 TB. olive oil

½ cup honey

1 TB. granulated sugar

1 tsp. salt

1 tsp. white pepper

3 cups red cabbage,
   shredded

1 head radicchio, shred-
   ded

1 cup red onion, sliced
   ⅛-inch thick

2 TB. chopped fresh basil

Each serving has:

84 calories

19 g carbohydrates

1 g fat

2 g fiber

1 g protein

1. Remove grape stems and cut each grape in ¹/₂.

2. Mix vinegar, olive oil, honey, sugar, salt, and pepper in a medium-to-large mixing bowl.

3. Add cabbage, radicchio, onions, chopped basil, and grapes. Toss until evenly covered.

4. Let stand in the refrigerator for 1 hour.

5. Remove from the refrigerator. Drain excess juice. Place slaw in a serving bowl. Serve.

Vivacious Violet Hummus with Veggies

Yield: 8 servings   *Prep time:* 15 minutes
Cook time: None   *Serving size:* ¼ cup

1 (15 oz.) can garbanzo beans, drained (reserve liquid)

2 TB. nonfat yogurt

3 cloves garlic, minced

1 tsp. ground cumin

Salt

½ tsp. black pepper

2 TB. lemon juice, fresh-squeezed

1 TB. extra-virgin olive oil

1 TB. tahini

½ cup beet juice

Celery sticks

Carrot sticks

Broccoli florets, slightly steamed

Red pepper strips

Each serving has:
229 calories
34 g carbohydrates
6 g fat
10 g fiber
11 g protein

1. In a large mixing bowl, combine garbanzo beans, yogurt, garlic, cumin, salt, pepper, lemon juice, olive oil, and tahini.

2. Place contents of the mixing bowl into a food processor. Blend on low speed. Gradually add beet juice and ¼ cup reserved garbanzo bean liquid, until desired consistency is reached.

3. Serve Vivacious Violet Hummus with celery, carrot, broccoli, and red pepper.

Cherry Clafoutis

Yield: 8 servings   *Prep time:* 10 minutes
Cook time: 30 minutes   *Serving size:* 1 slice

6 eggs

1¼ cups skim milk, warmed

6 TB. sugar

½ tsp. salt

¾ cup unbleached flour

2 cups cherries, pitted and chopped

Dash confectioner's sugar

Each serving has:
115 calories
24 g carbohydrates
1 g fat
1 g fiber
3 g protein

1. Preheat the oven to 400°F. Lightly grease a 9-inch round baking pan.

2. Combine eggs, milk, sugar, and salt in a food processor on low speed. Add in flour and blend well.

3. Lightly dust cherries with flour. Place fruit in the round baking dish.

4. Pour egg mixture over cherries.

5. Bake for 30 minutes or until a toothpick inserted into center of clafoutis comes out clean. Lightly dust with confectioner's sugar, and serve warm.

Pesto Chicken Salad with Red Grapes

Yield: 8 servings   *Prep time:* 10 minutes
Cook time: None; refrigerate 3 hours   *Serving size:* 6 ounces

¼ cup low-fat mayonnaise

2 TB. pesto sauce

1 tsp. lemon juice

1 TB. tarragon

Pinch sea salt

Dash white pepper

2 large eggs, hard-boiled and chopped

¾ lb. cooked chicken breast half, chopped

1 cup red grapes, halved

1 sprig fresh basil, chopped

Each serving has:
282 calories
9 g carbohydrates
14 g fat
1 g fiber
25 g protein

1. Combine mayonnaise, pesto sauce, lemon juice, tarragon, salt, and pepper in a bowl. Let stand.

2. In a separate bowl, mix eggs, chicken, grapes, and basil.

3. Combine dressing mixture with chicken mixture. Fold together.

4. Place in the refrigerator for at least 3 hours. Serve.

Cheesy Chakra Eggplant Omelet

Yield: 6 servings   *Prep time:* 10 minutes
Cook time: 10 minutes   *Serving size:* 1 omelet

2 cups Egg Beaters or 99 percent egg substitute

½ cup low-fat part-skim Mozzarella cheese, shredded

¼ cup low-fat Romano cheese, shredded

4 tsp. tomato, chopped

¼ cup water

4 TB. extra-virgin olive oil

1 large eggplant, peeled and sliced in ⅛-inch-thick slices

2 roasted red peppers, cut into strips

Salt and pepper

Each serving has:
164 calories
7 g carbohydrates
11 g fat
2 g fiber
10 g protein

1. In medium bowl, whisk together egg substitute, cheeses, tomato, and water. Set aside.

2. Place 4 tablespoons olive oil in a large nonstick skillet over medium-high heat. Sauté eggplant for 2 to 3 minutes on each side.

3. Add roasted peppers and sauté for 2 minutes.

4. Pour egg mixture over eggplant mixture.

5. Cook omelet on high heat, scrapping sides of pan constantly for 5 minutes or until eggs begin to stiffen.

6. When eggs have cooked completely use a spatula to fold and slide omelet onto serving dish.

7. Season with salt and pepper to taste and serve.

Baked Plum and Peach Delight

Yield: 6 servings   *Prep time:* 8 minutes
Cook time: 25 minutes   *Serving size:* 6 ounces

1½ cups plums, halved
1½ cups peaches, sliced
3 large eggs
¼ cup sugar

¼ cup whole-wheat flour
1 tsp. vanilla extract
2½ cups skim milk, warmed

Each serving has:
199 calories
27 g carbohydrates
7 g fat
2 g fiber
8 g protein

1. Preheat the oven to 375°F. Grease a 9-inch round pan with cooking spray.

2. Arrange plum halves and peach slices on the bottom of the pan.

3. In a large mixing bowl, combine eggs and sugar. Beat with a hand mixer on medium speed until smooth.

4. Add flour and vanilla. Beat for additional 3 minutes until well blended.

5. Gradually add in milk while beating with the mixer.

6. Pour batter over plums and peaches.

7. Bake for 25 to 30 minutes or until custard is golden. Serve warm or chilled.

Eggplant Mozzarella Wraps

Yield: 4 servings   *Prep time:* 8 minutes
Cook time: 5 minutes   *Serving size:* 1 wrap sandwich

4 whole-wheat tortillas	4 slices eggplant, grilled	*Each serving has:*
4 slices low-fat Mozzarella cheese	1 cup low-sodium marinara sauce	350 calories
		30 g carbohydrates
		15 g fat
		10 g fiber
		20 g protein

1. Preheat the oven to 375°F. Layer each tortilla with cheese, eggplant, and $1/4$ cup marinara sauce.

2. Place tortilla on a lightly greased cookie sheet. Bake in the oven for 5 minutes or until cheese melts and tortilla is lightly toasted. Serve warm.

Flaxseed Raisin Bread

Yield: 12 servings   *Prep time:* 10 minutes
Cook time: 55 minutes   *Serving size:* 1 slice

1½ cups whole-wheat flour
2 tsp. baking powder
¼ tsp. baking soda
1 tsp. salt
1¼ tsp. cinnamon
¼ tsp. nutmeg
1 cup packed dark brown
   sugar
1 cup rolled oats

1½ cups apple, peeled
   and grated
¼ cup walnuts, chopped
¼ cup raisins
2 eggs
3 TB. nonfat yogurt
2 TB. flaxseed oil
¼ cup skim milk
¼ cup vegetable oil

Each serving has:
224 calories
39 g carbohydrates
7 g fat
4 g fiber
4 g protein

1. Preheat the oven to 375°F. Grease and flour an 8¹/₂x4¹/₂-inch loaf pan.

2. In a large mixing bowl, combine flour, baking powder, baking soda, salt, cinnamon, nutmeg, dark brown sugar, and oats. Stir well. Gradually add apple, walnuts, raisins, eggs, yogurt, flaxseed oil, milk, and vegetable oil. Mix until well moistened.

3. Bake for 55 minutes or until a toothpick inserted in middle of loaf comes out clean. Cool completely prior to serving.

Spiced Red Cabbage, Apple, and Chestnut Salad

Yield: 4 servings   *Prep time:* 10 minutes
Cook time: 15 minutes   *Serving size:* 1 cup

1 large Vidalia onion, chopped fine

1 TB. extra-virgin olive oil

1 small red cabbage, shredded

5 large apples, chopped fine

¼ cup dark brown sugar

2 TB. red wine vinegar

½ tsp. salt

½ tsp. cinnamon

¼ tsp. allspice

½ cup water

½ cup golden seedless raisins

¼ cup roasted chestnuts

Each serving has:
279 calories
63 g carbohydrates
4 g fat
7 g fiber
2 g protein

1. In a large saucepan over medium-high heat, sauté onion in olive oil for 3 minutes or until translucent.

2. Add shredded cabbage and apples to the saucepan. Gradually add brown sugar, vinegar, salt, cinnamon, and allspice. Cook for 5 minutes over medium-low heat.

3. Add water. Simmer for 15 minutes or until cabbage is soft.

4. Remove from heat. Stir in onions and sprinkle with raisins and chestnuts.

5. Chill overnight and serve.

Gazpacho Salad

Yield: 4 servings   *Prep time:* 15 minutes
Cook time: None   *Serving size:* 1 cup

1 cup sliced celery

1 (15 oz.) can black beans, drained and rinsed

4 plum tomatoes, sliced ½-inch thick and halved

1 large yellow bell pepper

⅔ cup Chakra Salsa (recipe in Chapter 1)

⅓ cup nonfat sour cream

1 TB. lemon juice

3 TB. fresh cilantro, chopped

4 butter lettuce leaves, chopped

Each serving has:
398 calories
74 g carbohydrates
2 g fat
17 g fiber
25 g protein

1. Combine celery, black beans, tomatoes, and yellow peppers in a large bowl.

2. In a small bowl, combine salsa, sour cream, lemon juice, and cilantro. Pour contents of the small bowl over ingredients in the large bowl.

3. Toss well and serve portions over beds of lettuce.

Third-Eye Purple Sorbet

Yield: 4 servings   *Prep time:* 10 minutes
Cook time: None; freeze overnight   *Serving size:* 1 cup

1 cup plums, dried and pitted	32 oz. white grape juice, no sugar added	*Each serving has:*
6 TB. water, very hot		154 calories
1 TB. sugar	2 cups raspberries	38 g carbohydrates
2 TB. lemon juice, fresh-squeezed	½ cup blueberries	Trace fat
		4 g fiber
		1 g protein

1. In a blender or a food processor, combine plums with hot water. Process on medium speed until plums are chopped. Add sugar and lemon juice.

2. Gradually add grape juice, raspberries, and blueberries. Purée until very smooth.

3. Pour berry mixture into a shallow metal pan. Freeze overnight. Allow pan to stand 15 minutes prior to serving.

Purple Third-Eye Smoothie

Yield: 2 servings   *Prep time:* 10 minutes
Cook time: None   *Serving size:* 2 cups

1 large banana, peeled and sliced

½ cup blueberries

2 TB. flaxseed oil

1 TB. honey

½ tsp. vanilla extract

⅓ cup skim milk

½ cup nonfat yogurt

Each serving has:
156 calories
34 g carbohydrates
2 g fat
2 g fiber
6 g protein

1. Place banana, blueberries, flaxseed oil, honey, vanilla extract, milk, and yogurt in a blender, and purée.

2. Serve immediately.

Exercises to Balance Your Third-Eye Chakra

Let's get started with some personal-growth exercises that will balance your sixth energy center.

Get Forbidden Foods out of Your Line of Vision

The saying, "Out of sight, out of mind," is a good rule to remember when it comes to your diet. Eating healthy foods is extremely easy when you stock your home full of fresh, nutritious fruits and vegetables. This week, make every effort to make your home a safe and wholesome haven. Keep fresh fruit such as apples and bananas on the table in plain view. Make sure to keep ready-to-eat, healthy snacks, such as grapes and carrot sticks, at eye level in the refrigerator.

Make every effort to eliminate forbidden food temptations from your home. Clean out that pantry stuffed with brownie mix and Cheez Whiz. By allowing these items to remain in your house, you are setting yourself up for sabotage and failure. If you live with someone who absolutely insists upon keeping these foods in your home, ask that person to keep the food hidden from you.

Your sense of vision is an extremely powerful determinate to your behavior. Studies show that many smokers who go blind stop smoking cigarettes permanently after losing their vision. Commit to visualizing only healthy food in your home and workplace, to ensure your success.

Let Go of Your Old Story and Write a New One

Whether we are aware of it or not, we all see ourselves in a particular way. When we are healthy, our view of ourselves is typically positive and based in reality. When we carry excess weight and gorge on unhealthy foods, our self-esteem plummets and our perspective becomes pessimistic and distorted.

Clear your third-eye chakra by re-writing your life story and life script. Spend 20 minutes writing your current life story. After you write your existing story, attempt to create a new life script for yourself. Spend at least 30 minutes authoring your new life story. In your journal, ponder the following questions.

- What story do you currently tell yourself about your life?
- What roles do you play in your life now? What is your theme song?
- Do you see yourself as a perpetual victim who is always being taken advantage of? Are you always helping others and receiving nothing in return?
- What patterns or events constantly repeat themselves in your life?
- What will your new story be now that you have achieved permanent weight loss and feel peaceful?
- What is your new role in life? What can you offer yourself and others?

Write a Letter to Your Overweight Self from Your Thin Self

Write a letter from your formerly overweight, pessimistic self to your new healthy and positive self. You can date the letter 10 years from now, or 10 months from now, whatever feels right to you.

In your letter, reassure your overweight self that your new habits will lead to a happy, more fulfilled life. Tell your chubby self all about the lessons you learned while you were overweight and on your journey to thinness. Inform your fat self about all of the fun activities that you participate in now that you have healthy self-esteem and a trim physique.

Write about all the people, places, and things that you experience now that you are healthy and able to truly enjoy life. Talk about how refreshing it is to live in the moment in a state of joy. How do you spend your time now? What are your hopes and dreams? What advice can your overweight self offer to your skinny self? Pay attention to your own inner wisdom.

Write a Letter to Your Present-Day Self

For an even deeper experience, write a letter to your present-day self from yourself on your one-hundred-and-first birthday. Be kind and gentle with yourself in this missive. Tell your present-day self about all the life lessons you have learned and people you have touched during your time on Earth. Offer words of comfort, support, and encouragement. Talk about the adventures you have enjoyed over your many decades. Tell yourself precisely how you resolved some of your current struggles and problems. You will astound yourself, because much of the advice you give yourself can be implemented in your life right now to attain success and resolve crises.

Get Physical! Expand Your Vision Through Yoga

The Cat/Cow yoga pose is a beneficial tool to get energy flowing freely to your third-eye center. Known as Bidala/Gomukhuttanasana in Sanskrit, this posture stretches the muscles along your back, neck, and arms, and also promotes a sense of inner vision.

To begin this posture, take a few deep, cleansing breaths. Clear your mind of any cares or worries. Kneel in the table position. Form the table position by placing your knees under your hips. Keep your arms below your shoulders. Press your palms into the floor and keep your back straight. Take a few gentle breaths in table pose and relax.

On your next inhalation, slowly raise your head and tailbone simultaneously as you let your belly graze the floor. Allow your back to arch into a very subtle swayback position, taking great care not to overextend your spine. Look up toward the sky, without straining your neck. Yoga teacher Dawn Mehan encourages you to imagine that you are a gentle cow in a breezy pasture.

On your next exhalation, gently lower your head and your tailbone simultaneously. Arch your back, and continue to deeply exhale as you pull your navel up toward your spine. Imagine that you are a cat ready to pounce on the fun that life has to offer.

Continue to alternate between the cat and the cow positions, in sync with your breath. As you feel your energy begin to flow, decrease or increase these alternating movements in coordination with your breath. Continue this pose for three to five minutes, or for however long it feels comfortable for you.

Visualize Your Ideal Life and Body

Use your third-eye vision to create the body and life you have always desired. This week, make a collage or other concrete visual image of what you want to look like when you have attained your goal weight. Choose images from magazines, television, or even former photos of yourself. Select clothing, shoes, makeup, and hairstyles that you would wear if you were at your goal weight.

Post this picture in a place where you can see it daily and be reminded of your vision for the future. The refrigerator, bathroom mirror, and dashboard are all great places to display your vision collage with pride. This picture should make you feel inspired and joyous, not envious or resentful.

Make sure that these images are something you truly want for yourself, not things that other people desire for you. Place inspiring words or phrases on your vision collage to keep you motivated and excited about your goal. Each day, keep your eyes peeled for new things to add to your vision collage.

Envision Your "Do-Over"

We all have moments in our lives we wish we could do differently. Unfortunately, life does not always give us the opportunity to do things over. Perhaps you chose not to intervene while watching someone abuse her child or stole from your former employer. Or maybe you remained silent while someone touched you inappropriately or lashed out in anger at your own child. These moments cause you to feel bad about yourself and drain your psychic energy. These painful memories often keep you paralyzed in the past. They keep you stuck in an unhealthy body and mind that no longer serve you.

Take a few deep, cleansing breaths and gently close your eyes. Focus your energy and attention on your third-eye center. Think about the time in your life that you most want to "do over." Accept whatever memory comes forward. Do not dismiss the event or reject it as being trivial. Feel the emotions you experienced during this moment in time. Now imagine that you have been given the magical ability to go back in time and relive this moment. What would you do differently? How would it make you feel? Write about your experiences in your journal. Spend some time reflecting and sitting with your feelings. How can you use this experience to help yourself and others in the present?

Open Your Third-Eye and Reclaim Your Intuition

The third-eye chakra is closely associated with intuition and psychic powers. Medical research suggests that we humans only use a very small percentage of our brain. Engage all of the powers of your intellect this week by awakening the power of your intuitive mind. We all experience hunches but tend to dismiss them or second-guess their relevance. These little hunches can guide us to a healthy and peaceful lifestyle if they are heeded. Instead of dismissing your little hunches, pay close attention to them this week. In your journal, write about how you can use your sixth sense to create a slimmer body and healthier lifestyle.

Question Your Thoughts

Known as the center of concentration, your third-eye center directly reflects the thoughts in your mind. We tend to view our thoughts as something that happens to us, rather than a part of ourselves we can control and change for the better. For example, instead of gently noticing our thoughts, we become discouraged and depressed by them. The major reason thoughts are distressing is because we believe our thoughts are true.

Most of the time when we question our thoughts, we find that they are simply unfounded worries or anxious projections into the future or about the past. Most negative thinking proves to be speculative and a vain attempt to protect ourselves from disappointment. The next time you find yourself thinking a negative thought, immediately stop your thought process and begin questioning your mind. Ask yourself the following questions:

- Is this thought a true statement?

- Can I prove that this thought is actually true?

- How does this thought make me feel?
- How do I want to feel?
- What kind of thought feels better to me?

By continually asking yourself how your thoughts make you feel, you will become more aware of the direct connection between your thoughts and your emotions. Know that you have the power to change your thoughts and feel the way you choose. Instead of thinking the same old thoughts that cause you to feel forlorn and negative, try thinking new things that bring about feelings of passion and excitement. Replace antiquated, pessimistic thinking with fresh, hopeful thinking that makes you feel joyful.

Be Here Now: Learning to be Present with Yourself and Others

Most of us spend the majority of our time in our heads. Mental activities such as thinking, judging, rationalizing, and analyzing occupy most of our time. Instead of focusing on what we are doing in the present moment, we find ourselves rehashing past events or fretting about the future. When we are in a conversation with another person, we are so focused on formulating our response that we don't really listen to what our friend is saying to us. Some people focus so intensely on their partner that they lose track of their own needs and feelings in a conversation. Do either of these scenarios feel familiar to you? What is your personal pattern? Take some time to write about your experiences and patterns in your journal.

There are many ways of avoiding being in the present moment. The most common is spacing out or shutting down. Have you ever set out on a trip to the grocery store, only to arrive 20 minutes later and not remember any of the journey? Or have you ever sat down to watch a half-hour sitcom with a full bag of potato chips, and discover at the end of the program your bag is empty and you can't recall what the show was about? Chances are that you got lost in your own thoughts, or went on "automatic pilot."

Spacing out can be a beneficial emotional response when we need to relax after a long day at the office. The trouble is, for most people, spacing out becomes a way of life. Shutting down becomes a defense mechanism in early childhood. When young children become overwhelmed with feelings, and they are not taught how to deal with their emotions appropriately, they simply teach themselves to stop feeling. By habitually shutting down and stopping their emotions, people can become overweight, and struggle with a feeling of chronic emptiness. They can lose the pure ecstasy and peace that being in the present moment brings.

This week, practice being mindful when you are in dialogue with friends and family. Instead of attending to the dialogue inside your own head or engaging in self-talk, truly listen to what the other person is saying. Attempt to hear the tone and inflection in her voice. Perhaps your partner is saying polite words but his tone of voice is thick with contempt and sarcasm. Pay close attention to peoples' body language and posture. Are their words congruent with what their body is saying? For example, does your teenage daughter nod her head yes ever so slightly, as she screams the word no? Attempt to listen beyond words. You will find that you more deeply understand what your loved ones are attempting to communicate. If you feel yourself drifting off or becoming bored or disinterested during a conversation, find something in the present moment that excites or interests you. Perhaps your boredom is masking a deep-seated emotion that is calling out for your attention.

Most important, focus on your own inner experience. How do you hold your body when you are speaking? Do you fold your arms protectively across your solar plexus chakra? Do you frequently talk, and then cover your mouth with your hand as if to silence yourself?

In your journal, write about how you use your body when you communicate, and what this means to you. Make every effort to be present in all of your conversations this week. Focusing on your breathing is one surefire way to bring you into the present moment. Feeling your heartbeat within your chest is another technique to anchor your experience to the now. You will find that being present brings a sense of aliveness and joy to even difficult moments. Open yourself up to this experience now. Write about the experience in your journal.

Create a Serendipity Journal

Your third-eye chakra is your gateway to your own inner guidance and light. Life is a series of seemingly endless coincidences and serendipitous events. Perhaps you believe that these events are linked together by a divine source that guides your every move. Or perhaps you feel that life is a series of random, chaotic events with some lucky breaks intertwined.

Whatever you accept as true, pay close attention to any coincidences that show up in your life this week. For example, perhaps you are contemplating a move to Manhattan, and you inadvertently receive a copy of your neighbor's *New York Times* on your doorstep. Or maybe you are having a difficult time selling your house, when out of the blue an old friend calls to ask if you would consider selling your home to his son. These coincidences can offer us great clues to our life's purpose and direction.

Serendipitous events also can greatly enhance your weight-loss goals and sense of inner peace. For example, have you noticed how many healthy food selections you are offered now that you have committed yourself to this eating plan? Write about the coincidences you experience in your journal this week. What do these coincidences mean to you?

Another way to strengthen your third-eye chakra and overall sense of inner peace is to think of your entire life as a series of coincidences. In your journal, write about how your life has been linked by one serendipitous event after another. For example, how did you get your present job or meet your best friend? Write your life story and link all of these events together. How have you been led to where you are now? How has your entire life been leading up to this precise moment in time? How did this book find its way into your hands? How can you get from here to where you want to go in life? Pay close attention to the coincidences in your life this week; they will surely lead you to the life of your dreams.

7

Your Crown Chakra

The seventh chakra, or energy center, is located at the top of the head near the skull. This chakra represents spiritual enlightenment and union with the sacred and all living things. Your seventh energy center is associated with the colors white and violet. This week, wear white and violet clothing and gemstones to enhance your crown chakra.

Major issues signaling a blocked crown chakra include depression, apathy, lacking a sense of spirituality, or a fascination with religion or cults. When our seventh energy center is malfunctioning, we may feel disconnected from the flow of life, or depressed. Weight gain can cause us to isolate ourselves from our friends and loved ones. As a result, we experience a sense of vast loneliness and emptiness. We label ourselves as "different" and cut ourselves off from the joy of connecting with others and our higher self.

After completing this week's exercises, you will experience an enhanced sense of spiritual consciousness and connection with the universe. You were created to live the life you desire and fulfill your destiny. It is our intention that this chapter leads you to the inner peace that is always here for you in every moment.

Let's get started by taking a look at this week's eating plan.

CROWN CHAKRA SEVEN-DAY EATING PLAN

Day One

Breakfast: Gingerbread Waffles

Midmorning Snack: 1 large banana

Lunch: Better Than BLT Sandwich

Midafternoon Snack: $1/2$ cup pistachio nuts

Dinner: Mayan-Inspired Rice and Bean Casserole

Dessert: Peach Sorbet (recipe in Chapter 2)

Day Two

Breakfast: Date and Apricot Breakfast Bread and $1/2$ cup skim milk or soy milk

Midmorning Snack: 1 cup nonfat yogurt

Lunch: Chakra Tortilla Soup

Midafternoon Snack: 1 cup plain popcorn

Dinner: Penne Pasta with Spicy Artichoke Sauce

Dessert: Heavenly Chocolate Banana Popsicle (recipe in Chapter 3)

Day Three

Breakfast: Mushroom and Mozzarella Frittata

Midmorning Snack: 10 celery sticks and 2 tablespoons peanut butter

Lunch: Blissful Bean Salad

Midafternoon Snack: 1 hard-boiled egg

Dinner: Indian-Inspired Chicken Tikka Masala

Dessert: 1 cup nonfat yogurt with $1/2$ sliced banana

Day Four

Breakfast: Banana Chakra Smoothie

Midmorning Snack: $1/4$ cup almonds

Lunch: Seventh Chakra Grilled Ginger Cheese Sandwich

Midafternoon Snack: 1 cup plain popcorn

Dinner: Hugo's Inn Shiitake Mushroom Scampi

Dessert: Peach Sorbet (recipe in Chapter 2)

Day Five

Breakfast: Date and Apricot Breakfast Bread with $1/2$ cup skim milk or soy milk

Midmorning Snack: 1 small bunch seedless grapes

Lunch: Spanakopita Greek Salad

Midafternoon Snack: 10 carrot sticks

Dinner: Tilapia Casablanca

Dessert: $1/2$ cup sliced strawberries drizzled with skim milk

Day Six

Breakfast: Mushroom and Mozzarella Frittata

Midmorning Snack: 1 cup nonfat cottage cheese

Lunch: Cauliflower Cheese Nuggets

Midafternoon Snack: 1 hard-boiled egg

Dinner: Navajo Tacos

Dessert: Heavenly Chocolate Banana Popsicle (recipe in Chapter 3)

Day Seven

Breakfast: Gingerbread Waffles

Midmorning Snack: 1 slice Date and Apricot Breakfast Bread

Lunch: Grilled Mushrooms over Whole-Wheat Toast Points

Midafternoon Snack: $1/2$ cup almonds

Dinner: Mayan-Inspired Rice and Bean Casserole

Dessert: Peach Sorbet (recipe in Chapter 2)

Foods That Enhance Your Crown Chakra

Fruits and vegetables that contain white pigments and/or skins are excellent ways to support your seventh energy center and your overall health. Some fruits and vegetables with white or whitish pigments and skins include the following:

- Bananas
- Cauliflower
- Chives
- Garlic
- Leeks

- Mushrooms
- Parsnip
- Shallots
- Turnips

Crown Chakra Recipes

Here are this week's gourmet recipes that will enhance your crown chakra.

Cauliflower Cheese Nuggets

Yield: 4 servings   *Prep time:* 10 minutes
Cook time: 20 minutes   *Serving size:* 4 nuggets

2 cups cauliflower, fresh or
  frozen
1 cup whole-wheat bread-
  crumbs, seasoned

3 large eggs
1 cup cheddar cheese,
  shredded

Each serving has:
280 calories
22 g carbohydrates
8 g fat
4 g fiber
16 g protein

1. Heat the oven to 375°F.

2. Coat a baking sheet with vegetable oil spray and set aside.

3. In a large bowl, combine cauliflower, whole-wheat breadcrumbs, eggs, and cheese. Mix well.

4. Shape mixture into nuggets. Place on baking sheet approximately 3 inches apart.

5. Bake for 20 to 25 minutes, turning nuggets over after 15 minutes. Serve.

Indian-Inspired Chicken Tikka Masala

Yield: 4 servings   *Prep time:* 15 minutes; refrigerate 1 hour
Cook time: 30 minutes   *Serving size:* ¼-pound chicken with ½ cup sauce

1 cup nonfat yogurt

1 TB. lemon juice

4 tsp. ground cumin

1 tsp. ground cinnamon

⅛ tsp. cayenne

2 tsp. black pepper

1 TB. fresh ginger, minced

1 lb. chicken breast, boned, skinned, and cubed ¾-inches

2 TB. olive oil

1 TB. light butter

1 clove garlic, minced

1 small jalapeño pepper, chopped fine

2 tsp. paprika

8 oz. tomato sauce

1 cup skim milk

Dash salt

¼ cup fresh cilantro, chopped

Each serving has:
271 calories
15 g carbohydrates
11 g fat
2 g fiber
26 g protein

1. Combine yogurt, lemon juice, 2 teaspoons cumin, cinnamon, cayenne, black pepper, ginger, and chicken in a large bowl. Refrigerate for 1 hour.

2. Preheat a large skillet on medium-high heat. Add olive oil.

3. Sauté chicken about 15 minutes or until pink is gone, stirring constantly. Set chicken aside.

4. In a large heavy skillet, melt butter, and sauté garlic and jalapeño for 1 minute over medium heat.

5. Season with 2 teaspoons cumin and paprika.

6. Stir in tomato sauce and skim milk. Simmer on low for 20 minutes.

7. Add chicken. Simmer for 10 additional minutes.

8. Salt to taste, and garnish with cilantro.

Spanakopita Greek Salad

Yield: 10 servings   *Prep time:* 15 minutes
Cook time: 15 minutes   *Serving size:* 1½ cups

1 phyllo dough, sliced ½-
  inch thick

1 TB. anise seed

½ cup olive oil

4 cups iceberg lettuce leaf,
  torn

4 cups romaine lettuce leaf,
  torn

4 cups spinach leaves

2 tomatoes, cut into wedges

1 large cucumber, sliced

1 cup black pitted olives

3 TB. red wine vinegar

1 tsp. dried whole
  oregano

½ tsp. salt

½ tsp. ground pepper

1 cup feta cheese, crumbled

Each serving has:
287 calories
7 g carbohydrates
18 g fat
3 g fiber
5 g protein

1. Preheat the oven to 375°F.

2. Lay phyllo dough flat on a clean cutting surface. Mix anise seed with
   ¼ cup olive oil, and brush dough.

3. Cut dough into small triangles. Place triangles flat on a baking sheet.

4. Bake dough for 10 to 15 minutes. Remove from the oven and let cool.

5. Combine iceberg lettuce, romaine lettuce, spinach, tomatoes, cucumber, and olives in a large bowl. Toss well.

6. Combine additional ¼ cup olive oil, vinegar, oregano, salt, and pepper
   in a jar. Cover tightly and shake vigorously.

7. Toss salad with olive oil mixture just before serving. Place two baked
   phyllo triangles over salad, and sprinkle crumbled feta cheese overtop.

Date and Apricot Breakfast Bread

Yield: 16 servings   *Prep time:* 15 minutes
Cook time: 50 minutes   *Serving size:* 1 slice

1 cup dried apricots, chopped

2½ cups whole-wheat flour

1 cup sugar

3½ tsp. baking powder

1 tsp. cinnamon

1 tsp. salt

3 TB. butter, melted

½ cup skim milk

¾ cup orange juice

1 large egg, beaten

½ cup dates, chopped

½ cup walnuts, chopped

2 TB. orange zest

Each serving has:
203 calories
38 g carbohydrates
5 g fat
4 g fiber
5 g protein

1. Preheat the oven to 350°F. Lightly grease 2 standard loaf pans with vegetable cooking spray.

2. Place dried apricots in a small saucepan with 2 cups water. Heat until water boils. Allow to simmer for 5 minutes. Drain apricots and set aside.

3. In a large bowl, combine flour, sugar, baking powder, cinnamon, and salt. Stir until well blended.

4. Gradually stir in butter, milk, orange juice, and egg. Mix thoroughly.

5. Fold in dried apricots, dates, walnuts, and orange zest.

6. Place batter into loaf pans. Bake for 55 minutes or until a toothpick inserted into center of loaf comes out clean.

7. Cool and remove from the pan.

Seventh Chakra Grilled Ginger Cheese Sandwich

Yield: 2 servings   *Prep time:* 15 minutes
Cook time: None   *Serving size:* 1 sandwich

4 slices whole-grain bread, toasted

1 cup fat-free cream cheese

1 tsp. fresh ginger, grated

2 TB. honey

1 whole banana, sliced

Each serving has:
315 calories
58 g carbohydrates
5 g fat
7 g fiber
21 g protein

1. Toast bread slices.

2. Blend cream cheese, ginger, and honey until it has a smooth, spread-like consistency.

3. Evenly spread cheese on one side of each piece toast.

4. Place banana slices on one slice toast, and cover with other slice.

5. Slice in half. Serve.

Navajo Tacos

Yield: 8 servings   *Prep time:* 20 minutes
Cook time: 18 minutes   *Serving size:* 2 small tacos

½ cup canola oil

1 cup whole-wheat flour

1 cup all-purpose flour

2 TB. baking powder

¼ tsp. salt

¼ cup water

2 lb. ground turkey

1 onion, chopped fine

1 tsp. salt

1 tsp. garlic powder

2 Serrano chiles,
   chopped

2 (10 oz.) cans taco sauce

½ head lettuce

1 tomato, chopped small

½ lb. low-fat cheddar
   cheese, grated

Each serving has:
499 calories
29 g carbohydrates
28 g fat
5 g fiber
26 g protein

1. Preheat canola oil in a large 10-inch skillet on medium-high heat.

2. Mix flours, baking powder, and salt. Add enough water to make workable dough.

3. Pinch dough apart in 4 equal-size pieces.

4. Knead each piece 4 times. Roll out round to fit a 10-inch skillet.

5. Lay 1 piece at a time in the skillet with hot cooking oil.

6. Let fry until it bubbles, about 4 minutes. Turn over, and fry other side until golden brown.

7. Drain each bread piece on a paper towel. Place each one on a separate plate. Set aside.

8. Brown turkey meat in a pan with chopped onion, salt, and garlic powder.

9. When the meat is cooked, add Serrano chiles and taco sauce. Simmer for about 10 more minutes.

10. Spoon turkey mixture into dry bread. Top with lettuce, tomatoes, and cheddar cheese. Fold, and serve.

Penne Pasta with Spicy Artichoke Sauce

Yield: 6 servings   *Prep time:* 15 minutes
Cook time: 15 minutes   *Serving size:* 1½ cups

1 lb. whole-wheat penne pasta

3 TB. extra-virgin olive oil

4½ cup red onion, minced

1 TB. fresh garlic, minced

1 large banana pepper, chopped

1 cup tomatoes, chopped

8 oz. black olives, sliced

1 TB. Italian seasoning

1 tsp. red pepper flakes

Pinch kosher salt

8 oz. artichoke hearts, chopped

Each serving has:
422 calories
60 g carbohydrates
12 g fat
9 g fiber
13 g protein

1. Cook pasta according to package directions. Drain pasta in a colander and set aside.

2. In a large skillet, heat olive oil over medium-high heat.

3. Place onions, garlic, and banana peppers in the skillet. Cook for 3 to 5 minutes or until lightly browned.

4. Add tomatoes and olives. Cook for 5 more minutes.

5. Add Italian seasoning, red pepper flakes, salt, and artichokes. Simmer for 10 minutes, stirring occasionally.

6. Fold in pasta, until all pasta is coated with sauce. Serve.

Chakra Tortilla Soup

Yield: 12 servings   *Prep time:* 15 minutes
Cook time: 30 minutes   *Serving size:* 1½ cups

2 TB. extra-virgin olive oil

9 (6-inch) whole-wheat tortilla, cut into wedges

1 cup green onions, minced

1½ quarts long-grain brown rice

4 cups tomatoes, diced

2½ cups cooked chicken, cubed

1 cup whole-kernel corn, frozen, thawed (or use fresh)

1½ cups green chiles, chopped

3 quarts vegetable stock

3 TB. lime juice

¾ cup fresh cilantro, minced

12 lime slices

1½ cups diced avocado

Each serving has:
420 calories
61 g carbohydrates
12 g fat
6 g fiber
22 g protein

1. In a skillet over medium-high heat, heat 1 tablespoon olive oil. Fry tortilla wedges on both sides until golden and slightly crispy. Drain on paper towel. Set aside.

2. In a large saucepot, heat 1 tablespoon olive oil. Sauté green onions for 1 minute. Add rice, tomatoes, chicken, corn, chiles, and vegetable stock.

3. Bring to simmer. Cover. Cook on the stovetop for 15 minutes.

4. Stir in lime juice and tortilla wedges just prior to serving.

5. Garnish with cilantro, lime slices, and diced avocado. Serve.

Cauliflower Latkes

Yield: 4 servings   *Prep time:* 15 minutes
Cook time: 10 minutes   *Serving size:* 1 latke

1 large cauliflower, trimmed and cubed

1 medium onion, chopped fine

6 TB. canola oil

½ cup whole-wheat breadcrumbs, seasoned

¼ tsp. dried thyme

2 TB. parsley, minced

2 large eggs, lightly beaten

Salt and freshly ground pepper

½ cup fat-free sour cream, for dipping

Each serving has:
218 calories
12 g carbohydrates
12 g fat
2 g fiber
5 g protein

1. Steam cauliflower until very tender. Mash to consistency of mashed potatoes with ¼-inch lumps. Drain any excess moisture.

2. Heat 2 tablespoons oil over medium-low heat. Sauté onions until soft and lightly browned, about 10 minutes.

3. Combine mashed cauliflower, sautéed onions, breadcrumbs, thyme, parsley, eggs, salt, and pepper with a wooden spoon.

4. Heat 4 tablespoons oil in a deep skillet.

5. Scoop out heaping tablespoon of cauliflower mixture into your hands. Compress into patty about ¹/₂-inch thick.

6. Place patty in hot oil to fry. Repeat with remaining cauliflower, cooking 4 to 5 patties at a time, flipping when golden on the first side. Do not crowd pan or they will not brown and crisp properly.

7. Drain cauliflower latke on paper towels. Keep warm in the oven at 250°F until all are completed. Serve with fat-free sour cream for dipping.

Better Than BLT Sandwich

Yield: 2 servings   *Prep time:* 15 minutes
Cook time: 10 minutes   *Serving size:* 1 sandwich

2 large portobello mush-
  rooms, grilled

2 TB. low-fat sour cream

4 large lettuce leaves

3 large fresh basil leaves,
  chopped

2 pinches salt

2 pinches black pepper

4 slices tomatoes

4 slices whole-grain
  bread, toasted

Each serving has:
380 calories
70 g carbohydrates
7 g fat
18 g fiber
20 g protein

1. Grill mushrooms until soft in middle, about 5 minutes each side. Cool for 10 minutes.

2. Spread sour cream evenly on all 4 slices bread.

3. Place lettuce leaves and tomato on 2 slices bread.

4. Sprinkle chopped basil, salt, and pepper over tomatoes.

5. Place mushrooms on top of tomatoes.

6. Cover with remaining slices bread. Serve.

Grilled Mushrooms over Whole-Wheat Toast Points

Yield: 4 servings   *Prep time:* 15 minutes
Cook time: 15 minutes   *Serving size:* 2 slices

3 large portobello mush-
rooms

1 clove garlic, minced

1 tsp. black pepper

1 tsp. onion powder

½ cup olive oil

2 oz. sherry vinegar

Dash kosher salt

1 can cream of mush-
room soup, fat-free

8 slices whole-grain
bread

2 pinches parsley

Each serving has:
385 calories
48 g carbohydrates
16 g fat
7 g fiber
11 g protein

1. In a small bowl, combine portobello mushrooms, garlic, black pepper, onion powder, olive oil, sherry vinegar, and salt. Set aside to marinate.

2. Prepare mushroom soup as per directions on the can. Keep warm on the stove.

3. Toast bread and slice into triangles. Arrange toast points on a serving plate.

4. Remove mushrooms from marinade. Discard marinade. Grill whole portabellos for about 5 minutes on each side or until soft in the middle. Remove from heat and slice ¼-inch thick.

5. Place sliced grilled portobellos over toast points. Pour soup over the entire dish. Garnish with parsley.

Mushroom and Mozzarella Frittata

Yield: 4 servings   *Prep time:* 15 minutes
Cook time: 15 minutes   *Serving size:* 6 ounces

4 TB. canola oil

2 TB. fat-free sour cream

1 tsp. onion powder

Dash salt

Dash black pepper

6 whole organic eggs, beaten

1 large portobello mushroom, sliced ½-inch thick

½ cup shiitake mushroom, sliced ⅓-inch thick

¼ cup onions, diced fine

¼ cup red and green bell pepper, diced fine

¼ cup Mozzarella cheese, shredded

Each serving has:
310 calories
28 g carbohydrates
15 g fat
4 g fiber
15 g protein

1. Preheat the oven to 375°F degrees.

2. Place canola oil in a large, oven-proof skillet. Preheat on the stovetop over medium-high heat.

3. Whisk sour cream, onion powder, salt, and pepper into eggs until all sour cream is incorporated into eggs.

4. Place mushrooms, onions, and peppers into the skillet. Cook for 3 to 5 minutes, stirring constantly.

5. Place eggs into the skillet. Cook for 1 to 2 minutes, continually stirring. Continue to stir until eggs become firm. Remove from heat.

6. Sprinkle Mozzarella cheese on top of frittata. Place in the oven. Cook for 10 to 15 minutes.

7. Remove from the oven. Let stand for 3 minutes.

8. Run a plastic spatula around edge of the skillet to loosen eggs. Slide frittata onto a cutting board. Slice into 4 equal triangles. Serve with a dollop of sour cream.

Hugo's Inn Shiitake Mushroom Scampi

Yield: 4 servings   *Prep time:* 15 minutes
Cook time: 15 minutes   *Serving size:* 6 ounces

2 cups brown rice, cooked

¼ cup olive oil

2 TB. garlic, minced

¼ cup red onion, minced

2 cups shiitake mushroom, sliced, stems removed

1 TB. lemon juice

¼ cup white wine

1 TB. fresh basil, chopped

Dash salt

Dash white pepper

Each serving has:
601 calories
72 g carbohydrates
15 g fat
15 g fiber
21 g protein

1. Preheat 3 tablespoons olive oil in a large skillet over medium-high heat.

2. Add garlic, onions, and shiitake mushrooms. Cook for 2 to 5 minutes, stirring constantly.

3. When mixture begins to brown, add lemon juice and remaining oil. Continue to cook for 4 minutes. Gradually add white wine.

4. Let mixture cook, until reduced by about a fourth.

5. Stir in fresh basil, salt, and pepper. Remove from heat. Let stand 3 minutes.

6. Serve over hot, cooked rice.

Blissful Bean Salad

Yield: 4 servings   *Prep time:* 15 minutes
Cook time: 4 minutes   *Serving size:* 1½ cups

1½ cups edamame beans, shelled	Pinch salt	*Each serving has:*
	Dash black pepper	129 calories
2 cups cherry tomatoes	1 TB. olive oil	12 g carbohydrates
1 cup cucumber, sliced	2 TB. Balsamic vinegar	7 g fat
½ cup red onion, chopped	16 bibb lettuce leaves	4 g fiber
		7 g protein

1. To cook edamame, bring 3 cups salted water to a boil.

2. Add shelled edamame and cook 4 minutes.

3. Drain and rinse with cold running water to cool.

4. In a large bowl, combine cherry tomatoes, cucumber, onion, edamame beans, salt, pepper, oil, and vinegar.

5. Toss well. Serve bean mixture over bed of bibb lettuce.

Tilapia Casablanca

Yield: 4 servings   *Prep time:* 1 hour
Cook time: 20 minutes   *Serving size:* ¼ pound

2 tsp. paprika

1 tsp. ground cumin

1 tsp. ground ginger

1 tsp. turmeric

½ tsp. cinnamon

¼ tsp. black pepper, fresh-ground

1 lb. tilapia

3 TB. olive oil

Salt, to taste

3 cloves garlic, minced

1 onion, chopped

Peel from 1 lemon, rinsed in cold water, cut into thin strips

1 cup green olives, pitted

½ cup golden seedless raisins

¼ cup water

¼ cup parsley, chopped

¼ cup cilantro, chopped

Each serving has:
292 calories
23 g carbohydrates
11 g fat
3 g fiber
25 g protein

1. Combine paprika, cumin, ginger, turmeric, cinnamon, and pepper in a small bowl.

2. Pat tilapia fillets dry. Coat well with spice mixture. Let tilapia stand in spices for 1 hour in the refrigerator.

3. In a large, heavy-bottomed skillet, heat 2 tablespoons olive oil on medium-high heat. Add tilapia pieces, and sprinkle lightly with salt. Brown in the skillet, skin side down, for 5 minutes.

4. Lower heat to medium-low. If needed, add 1 tablespoon olive oil. Add garlic and onions. Cover and let cook for 5 minutes.

5. Turn tilapia fillets over. Add lemon peel slices, olives, raisins, and ¹/₄ cup water. Bring to a simmer on medium heat, and cook for an additional 5 minutes.

6. Mix in fresh parsley and cilantro right before serving. Adjust seasonings to taste. Serve.

Mayan-Inspired Rice and Bean Casserole

Yield: 4 servings   *Prep time:* 15 minutes
Cook time: 30 minutes   *Serving size:* 2 cups

⅓ cup fat-free yogurt

3 TB. cilantro, chopped

½ cup Chakra Salsa (recipe in Chapter 1)

½ cup green onion, sliced

½ cup red and green bell pepper, chopped

5 garlic cloves, minced

Dash white wine

2 cups whole-kernel corn

1 cup tomato, chopped

1 cup brown rice, cooked

½ cup olives

1 medium zucchini sliced

2 cups black beans

Each serving has:
511 calories
90 g carbohydrates
4 g fat
19 g fiber
30 g protein

1. Preheat the oven to 350°F.

2. Mix yogurt, cilantro, and Chakra Salsa. Set aside.

3. Cut onion slices in half; sauté onions, red peppers, green peppers, and garlic in wine until soft.

4. Lightly coat a casserole dish with nonstick vegetable spray, then layer corn, tomatoes, rice, olives, zucchini, sautéed onions, and beans.

5. Cover and cook 30 minutes or until thoroughly heated. Serve.

Whole-Wheat Vegetable Bruschetta

Yield: 6 servings   *Prep time:* 15 minutes
Cook time: 10 minutes   *Serving size:* 1 slice

1 whole-wheat bread loaf, sliced in half horizontally

1 medium zucchini, diced fine

1 medium summer squash, diced fine

2 medium ripe tomatoes, chopped small

1 medium red onion, diced fine

½ cup fresh basil, chopped

2 TB. olive oil

2 TB. garlic, minced

3 TB. Balsamic vinegar

Dash salt

Dash ground black pepper

3 cups Mozzarella cheese, shredded

Each serving has:
278 calories
13 g carbohydrates
16 g fat
3 g fiber
15 g protein

1. Preheat the oven to 400°F.

2. Place halved bread loaf on a cookie sheet.

3. In a large bowl, mix zucchini, squash, tomatoes, and onions. Set aside.

4. In a medium bowl, mix basil, olive oil, garlic, vinegar, salt, and pepper.

5. Lightly brush exposed side of bread with oil mixture.

6. Combine remaining oil mixture with vegetables. Mix well.

7. Top bread evenly with vegetable mixture.

8. Place Mozzarella cheese on top vegetable mixture.

9. Bake in the oven for 10 minutes or until cheese melts. Remove and slice. Serve.

Gingerbread Waffles

Yield: 9 servings   *Prep time:* 15 minutes
Cook time: 5 minutes   *Serving size:* 1 waffle

¾ cup all-purpose flour

1 cup whole-wheat flour

2 tsp. baking powder

½ tsp. cinnamon

½ tsp. salt

1½ TB. sugar

3 whole organic eggs

6 TB. canola oil

1 tsp. ginger, fresh-
ground

1½ cups skim milk

Fat-free yogurt

Each serving has:

212 calories

22 g carbohydrates

11 g fat

2 g fiber

6 g protein

1. Preheat the waffle iron.

2. Sift flours, baking powder, cinnamon, salt, and sugar into a medium-
   size bowl.

3. Separate eggs, putting egg whites in a smaller bowl. Beat egg whites
   until stiff.

4. Add egg yolks, oil, ginger, and milk to dry ingredients. Beat until there
   are no lumps in batter.

5. Fold egg whites into other batter using a spatula or another flat utensil.
   Put ¹/₂ cup batter in a waffle iron to make a 9-inch round waffle.

6. Garnish waffle with a dollop of fat-free yogurt. Serve.

Exercises to Balance Your Crown Chakra

Let's get started with some personal-growth exercises that will balance your seventh energy center.

Get In Touch with Your Greatest Prejudice

This week, be courageously honest with yourself about the assumptions you make about other people. In your journal, write about the following questions and statements.

- What groups do you prefer not to interact with?

- If you are brutally honest, what particular races, cultures, creeds, ethnicities and/or religions annoy you? Identify what it is that disturbs you.

- What feelings does this particular group stir within you?

- Do you see a part of yourself in the group you dislike? You will likely find that you are projecting the most disliked parts of yourself onto this group. Understand that the prejudices you hold are not really about the group you dislike, but rather about yourself.

- This week, vow to learn something about the group that you dislike the most. Attempt to get to know a person from this culture.

- How is your own culture more alike than different from this culture?

Celebrate Multicultural Style!

Hundreds of cultures have much to teach us about eating properly and nourishing our bodies. Every week or month, have a multicultural celebration night in your home. Here are some suggestions for celebrating and embracing other cultures:

- Prepare a healthy recipe indigenous of another tradition.

- Enhance your cultural experience by playing traditional music or watching a film about a country and/or its people.

- Give each family member an opportunity to select and research a culture.

- Invite people of other races, ethnicities, and religions into your home to celebrate with you.

Watch Your Life Like a Play

A great way to align your seventh chakra and achieve inner peace is to watch your life like a play. Attempt to view the inner and outer circumstances of your life like a curious and detached theatergoer. Endeavor to take things less personally, and pay more attention to what is going on in the moment. Learn how to do this by responding to the following questions and statements:

- How does it feel to observe your life with a sense of detachment? Do you notice your sense of wonder and serenity increasing as you gain clarity about your life's purpose?

- How can you use your newfound sense of awareness to achieve your weight-loss goals?

- Notice all of the characters in your life's play. Who is the main character in your play? Are you the main character in your own life or does it revolve around the behavior of your child or partner?

- What is your main character's biggest obstacle? Who is the true antagonist in the story line? What are the main life lessons and patterns of behavior in the play?

- What have you learned by watching your life like a play?

Lose Your Ego and Find Your True Self

Your ego is a part of your personality that barks orders at you in the form of self-talk. It is that nagging voice inside your head that constantly tells you what you should and ought to do. Your ego tries to convince you that you need to meet certain conditions before you can be happy. For example, your ego dictates that you will be satisfied only when you lose 10 pounds. However, once you drop the 10 pounds, your ego will form a new desire and a new condition for happiness.

It is firmly focused on the future or the past. "When you retire, then you can pursue you dreams," the ego taunts. Know that your ego never wants you to experience the joy in the present moment. The ego's primary role and function is to elude satisfaction and inner peace. Your ego always will want more, and will encourage you to postpone happiness and inner peace until certain conditions are met.

This week, learn to tame your ego by refusing to adhere to its endless demands. Decide that you will experience peace and happiness (or whatever your desired state) right now. Happiness and inner peace are always here for you. You just need to let yourself experience the feelings. You can enjoy the great outdoors and the warm sun on your face, regardless of whether you are living in a homeless shelter in Los Angeles or residing in a Malibu mansion.

In your journal, write about what your ego currently is demanding of you in this moment. How can you release this demand, and experience the freedom and inner peace you desire?

Get Physical! Exercises to Open Your Crown Chakra

The Downward Facing Dog yoga pose increases energy and blood circulation to your crown chakra center. In addition, it greatly improves mental clarity and concentration. Also known as Adho Mukhasana in Sanskrit, this pose releases tension in the shoulders, and also helps promote a sense of connection to the universe.

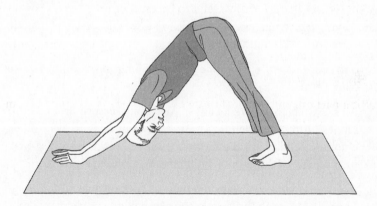

Downward Facing Dog

To begin this posture, take a few deep, cleansing breaths. Clear your mind of any thoughts. Kneel in the table position. The table position is formed by placing your knees under your hips. Keep your arms below your shoulders. Press your palms into the floor and keep your back straight. Take a few gentle breaths in table pose and relax.

On your next inhalation, tuck your toes under, as you lift your buttocks toward the sky. Take care to keep your knees slightly bent and engage your core muscles.

On your next exhalation, push your palms down into the floor. Align your chest with your thighs. Imagine that you are pressing your chest deeply toward your thighs. Release all tension in your neck and shoulders. Breathe deeply in and out for three deep, cleansing breaths. Welcome everything you are experiencing right now.

On your fourth inhalation, raise your left heel. Keep your right foot firmly planted on the floor. Make sure that your right leg is straight and grounded to the earth. On your next exhalation, return your left leg to the floor and raise your right heel. Alternate raising and lowering your heels for two minutes or until your body needs to rest. As you finish the pose, offer gratitude for your strong body and connection to all living things.

See Yourself in Everyone

Being unhappy with your weight is a very isolating experience. When we are dissatisfied with the way we look or feel, we disconnect from the deeper adventures life offers. We tend to become absorbed in our own thoughts, lives, and struggles. As a result, we lose sight of the connection that we share with all living beings.

Learn to see yourself in everyone by responding to the following questions in your journal:

- All human beings have feelings. We feel joy, ecstasy, grief, and sadness. Although the mechanisms of our injuries are diverse, our emotional and physical pain are the same. How is your personal pain similar to the pain of a billionaire or a homeless person?

- This week, view everyone you meet as your own daughter or son. Instead of judging the surly cashier or belligerent client, try to see the small child that exists within her. Recognize that angry or contemptuous behavior is often a defense mechanism used to hide feelings of shame and disconnection. What do you notice when you observe other's behavior in this way?

- Rather than argue or attempt to convince others that you are right, strive to be compassionate. Make every effort to distract yourself and others from pain by focusing on the positive aspects of a situation. How does it feel when you let go of your need to be right or be in control of every situation?

🕸 Spend one entire day this week viewing all people and things in nature as if they were a part of you. When you look into the eyes of your neighbor, boss, and mother-in-law, see your own inner reflection staring back at you. What is the common ground that unites you with others?

🕸 Try to remove all labels that you place on yourself. Our tendency to put ourselves in categories limits our potential and disengages us from the rest of the world. What labels do you place upon yourself and how do these roles lock you in a position that inhibits your personal growth?

🕸 Write what you have in common with the following individuals: a heroin addict, a millionaire, a supermodel, an autistic child, and a monk. How is everyone you meet a part of you?

Share Your Secret: Set Your Skeletons Free

We all carry a secret, a part of ourselves that we attempt to hide from those around us at all costs. This secret causes us so much shame that the mere thought of revealing it brings about intense feelings of anxiety and dread. This secret drains a large quantity of our energy from our seventh chakra and depletes our sense of self-worth. Feelings of unworthiness and shame keep us feeling separate and isolated from others.

In your journal, write about your secret and how it has impacted your life. How does your secret keep you stuck in the past, and trapped in an unhealthy body and mind? Find a trusted friend, professional counselor, or clergyperson, and tell her your secret. You will find that when you unload the secret, you will also lose pounds.

Connecting to Everything Through Meditation

Find a comfortable place to sit and meditate. Ideally, this place will be outdoors in nature. However, this meditation can be just as beneficial if it is practiced indoors. Be sure to choose a location that works for you in your life right now.

Gently close your eyes and take a few deep, cleansing breaths. Clear your mind of any thoughts or worries. Welcome everything you are experiencing right now. As thoughts, feelings, and sounds arise, simply notice them and let them go. Allow these thoughts, feelings, and noises to deepen your state of relaxation and meditation, instead of disturbing it.

Sit with your back straight and your head held high. Rest your hands on your knees, with your palms facing upward toward the sky. Gently press your thumbs to your index fingers. This way of sitting will help get the energy flowing to all seven of your chakra centers.

As you begin, either silently or aloud, state your intention for this meditation. "I intend to connect with all living things in the universe. I will see myself in everyone and everything I encounter today."

Either silently or aloud, begin chanting the word "OM." Allow your attention to remain on your breathing and the word OM. OM is the sound of love. OM is the divine sound that connects all living things in the world. OM is a sound that we share with the oceans, the trees, and all living beings. If you listen closely, you will notice that this sound is present in everything that surrounds you.

Can you feel your hands vibrating as you chant OM? That tickling sensation you feel is the love energy you share with everything and everyone in the universe. Know that this energy is always here waiting for you. You have the power to summon this energy anywhere and anytime. When you feel stressed and tempted to overeat, you can always tap into this source. Simply close your eyes and focus on the word OM as you pay attention to your breath and bodily sensations.

When you are ready, end this meditation by giving thanks for the life energy that supports you in every movement. Attempt to carry the feeling of love and connectedness with you, and bring it to every person you encounter today.

Embracing Opposites

Life is full of ups and downs. It is a series of events that we react to by feeling either good or bad about what we observe. Most of our reactions to life are conditioned responses. For example, many people associate rain with gloomy moods, messy driving, and canceled activities. But just watch a toddler dance happily in a rain puddle, and you will notice that the small child delights in what many adults find troublesome.

We learn to associate specific events with certain feelings and behaviors. How many of your thoughts and feelings are really your own? Or are you simply reacting to events as you were taught? How do you try to dictate and control the feelings and experiences of those around you? This week, give yourself and those around you permission to truly have their own feelings and experiences.

Think back on your life and remember the times when you felt the most joy and happiness. Now reflect on your life, as you recall the moments that brought you the greatest sadness and fear. Write about these moments in your journal. It is in your nature to embrace moments of joy and happiness, and to resist moments of grief and sadness. This week, notice your reaction to events around you and the emotional responses they awaken within you.

Instead of pushing away feelings of discomfort or sadness, welcome these feelings, and be open to what they have to teach you. A good way to begin this process is simply labeling what you are experiencing, and setting a timer for five minutes. Give yourself permission to focus fully on your feelings for five minutes. Spend as much time as you need, sitting with your feelings and noticing what is happening in your body. Remember to fully experience the joy that shows up in your life.

Know that sadness and joy are two opposite ends of the spectrum, but are both equally important experiences. Keep in mind that everything in life exists on a continuum. The best things in life are rarely in black or white, but rather in shades of gray. When you are trying to lose weight, it's easy to think in terms of either "fat" or "thin." This week, learn to embrace every aspect of yourself during your journey from fat to thin. Enjoy all of the feelings, encounters, and clothing sizes of your experience, on your road to healthy, peaceful living.

Find a Power Greater Than Yourself

In modern American culture, there is a strong emphasis on individualism and independence. People in our society take great pride in harnessing personal power and making a name for themselves. Although achievement and independence are laudable values, they often leave us feeling isolated and cut off from a sense of spirituality. Read the following questions and statements and write about your thoughts and feelings.

✺ This week, endeavor to discover a power greater than yourself. Many people choose to call this power God and connect with this force through prayer or meditation. Others find a power greater than themselves in nature by walking in a forest or floating along the ocean in a sailboat. What power greater than yourself do you easily connect with?

- Many recovering alcoholics and addicts find a power greater than themselves in the rooms where 12-step meetings are held. Others simply turn their problems over to the universe. How can you use a power greater than yourself to resolve the issues in your life that you perceive as problems?

- This power can be an invaluable resource when you are struggling with weight loss and living a healthy lifestyle. What specific things can you count on to help you reconnect with this power when you need help? Religious relics, scripture verses, quotes, or uplifting friends are just a few ways to access this power.

- What places feel sacred to you and help you feel the presence of a power greater than yourself? Do you feel most connected to this power in a synagogue, a church, in your own backyard, or in a foreign land? If you don't have the time, money, or energy for travel now, read about these places and imagine how it would feel to visit them.

8

Your Entire Chakra System: The Rainbow Within

Congratulations! You have reached the end of this book and the beginning of a new journey. Be proud of your accomplishments and your intention to create a healthy body, mind, and spirit. You have worked hard to lose weight and attain serenity. Remember that your intention to change your life is a powerful force that has the ability to transform your life forever. True inner peace requires no next step, exercise, or recipe. It is already here. It exists within you at all times. Accessing it is simply a matter of tapping into your own inherent wisdom.

This chapter contains recipes and personal-growth exercises that will help you to maintain the good eating and personal-growth habits you acquired. This of the book has a myriad of recipes that contain fruits and vegetables to stimulate all of the chakras. In addition, there are personal-growth exercises that will help you maintain and deepen your sense of inner stillness and peace.

There are many different ways to incorporate the Inner Peace Diet into your daily life. Some people decide to repeat weeks one though seven of the diet consecutively for a whole year or longer. Others pick and choose eating plans based on their personal needs. For example, a person struggling with survival and financial issues may focus on chapter one for several weeks, while a person struggling with spirituality may spend an entire season doing the exercises in chapter seven. Other clients prepare one Inner Peace Diet weekly for their family and spend dinnertime discussing that particular chakra. There is no right or wrong way to use this book. Enjoy every step on your ongoing journey in health and happiness.

The creators of *The Inner Peace Diet* offer several East Coast retreats each year, in addition to individual and group life-coaching services. To gain a deeper understanding of yourself and learn more about our programs, please visit www.innerpeacediet.com.

Rainbow Recipes for Your Entire Being

Here are some gourmet recipes that will enhance all seven of your major chakras.

Rainbow Ratatouille

Yield: 6 servings   *Prep time:* 15 minutes
Cook time: 20 minutes   *Serving size:* 1 cup

1 large eggplant, sliced into 1-inch-thick rounds

1 large yellow bell pepper, diced

1 large red bell pepper, diced

3 TB. extra-virgin olive oil

6 cloves garlic, minced

2 (14 oz.) cans diced tomatoes

1 (16 oz.) can chickpeas, drained and rinsed

Salt and pepper

½ cup fresh basil, chopped

Each serving has:
404 calories
61 g carbohydrates
12 g fat
18 g fiber
18 g protein

1. Place eggplant on a lightly oiled baking sheet. Broil eggplant for 5 minutes or until golden brown.

2. Turn over eggplant. Broil other side for additional 3 minutes.

3. Remove from the pan and set aside.

4. In a stockpot, heat olive oil over medium-high heat. Sauté garlic and peppers for 5 minutes or until lightly golden.

5. Add tomatoes to the stockpot. Simmer for 10 minutes. Add chickpeas and peppers. Stir.

6. Season with salt and pepper to taste. Cut eggplant into small dices. Gently stir in eggplant and basil. Serve.

Rainbow Pasta Primavera

Yield: 6 servings   *Prep time:* 15 minutes
Cook time: 60 minutes   *Serving size:* 1 cup

2 TB. extra-virgin olive oil

2 cloves garlic, chopped

4½ oz. diced tomatoes

6 oz. tomato paste

1 cup broccoli florets

1 cup carrot, sliced thin

¾ cup Vidalia onion

½ cup zucchini, sliced 1-inch thick

½ cup red pepper, chopped coarse

½ cup green bell pepper, chopped coarse

2 bay leaves

2 TB. fresh basil, minced

½ tsp. dried oregano

½ tsp. rosemary

½ tsp. thyme

½ tsp. sugar

⅓ cup water

2 tsp. salt

1½ lb. hot, cooked whole-wheat pasta

Each serving has:
487 calories
90 g carbohydrates
4 g fat
13 g fiber
19 g protein

1. In a large saucepot over medium heat, add 1 tablespoon olive oil and sauté garlic for 3 minutes. Gradually add diced tomatoes, tomato paste, broccoli, carrots, onion, zucchini, red pepper, green pepper, and bay leaves to saucepot.

2. Heat to a boil and simmer uncovered for 5 minutes.

3. Add 1 tablespoon olive oil, basil, oregano, rosemary, thyme, sugar, water, and salt. Reduce heat to low, and cover.

4. Cook for approximately 5 minutes, or until vegetables are tender.

5. Pour sauce over whole-wheat pasta and serve.

Multigrain Pancakes with Fresh Fruit Salsa

Yield: 4 servings   *Prep time:* 10 minutes
Cook time: 10 minutes   *Serving size:* 2 small pancakes

½ cup all-purpose flour

½ cup whole-wheat flour

¼ cup quick-cooking oats

2 TB. cornmeal, whole-grain

2 TB. brown sugar

1½ tsp. baking powder

½ tsp. salt

1 cup skim milk

¼ cup nonfat yogurt

1 large egg

Each serving has:
237 calories
38 g carbohydrates
6 g fat
3 g fiber
9 g protein

1. In a large bowl, combine all-purpose flour, whole-wheat flour, quick-cooking oats, cornmeal, brown sugar, baking powder, and salt. Mix well.

2. Gradually add milk, yogurt, and egg. Stir until smooth.

3. Spoon ¹/₄ cup batter onto a hot nonstick griddle or skillet coated with nonstick vegetable cooking spray over medium-high heat.

4. Cook pancake for 2 minutes or until edges are golden. Turn pancake over. Cook for 2 additional minutes or until bubbles form on top, and edges are brown. Serve with Fresh Fruit Salsa.

Fresh Fruit Salsa

Yield: 4 servings   *Prep time:* 15 minutes
Cook time: None; refrigerate 2 hours   *Serving size:* 1 cup

1 cup strawberries, diced

1 large peach, pitted and diced

1 cup kiwifruit, diced

1 large apple, cored and diced

2 TB. lemon juice

¼ cup dark brown sugar

¼ tsp. nutmeg

½ tsp. cinnamon

Each serving has:
141 calories
36 g carbohydrates
1 g fat
4 g fiber
1 g protein

1. In a large bowl, combine strawberries, peach, kiwi, and apple.

2. Gently stir in lemon juice, brown sugar, nutmeg, and cinnamon. Stir well.

3. Refrigerate for 2 hours. Serve.

Spinach "Lasagna" with Rainbow Veggies

Yield: 6 servings   *Prep time:* 15 minutes
Cook time: 40 minutes   *Serving size:* 1½ cups

10 oz. spinach, frozen, chopped

1 lb. lean ground turkey

1 (15 oz.) can low-sodium tomato sauce

1 tsp. sugar

½ tsp. salt

2 cloves garlic, minced

⅛ tsp. black pepper

½ cup red bell pepper, coarsely chopped

½ cup green bell pepper, coarsely chopped

3 cups whole-wheat egg noodles, cooked and drained

1 (8 oz.) package low-calorie cream cheese, softened

½ cup nonfat sour cream

3 TB. skim milk

2 TB. onions, chopped fine

½ cup fat-free cheddar cheese

Each serving has:
346 calories
29 g carbohydrates
13 g fat
4 g fiber
27 g protein

1. Preheat the oven to 350°F. Cook spinach according to package directions. Drain spinach on a paper towel.

2. In a large skillet coated with nonstick vegetable cooking spray cook ground turkey until browned. Drain off fat.

3. In the large skillet with ground turkey, stir in tomato sauce, sugar, salt, garlic, black pepper, red and green peppers, and noodles. Set aside.

4. In a medium bowl, combine cream cheese, sour cream, milk, and onion.

5. In a 2-quart casserole dish coated with nonstick vegetable spray, layer in the following order: ¹/₂ ground-turkey mixture, all the spinach, ¹/₂ cream cheese mixture, and remaining ground-turkey mixture.

6. Bake covered for 40 minutes.

7. Uncover dish. Sprinkle with cheddar cheese. Bake uncovered for additional 7 minutes or until cheese melts. Serve.

Rainbow Fruit Pizza

Yield: 12 servings   *Prep time:* 10 minutes
Cook time: 10 minutes   *Serving size:* 1 slice

½ cup margarine

½ cup sugar

2 tsp. cinnamon

2 tsp. vanilla extract

1 large egg

2 cups whole-wheat flour

2 tsp. baking powder

1 (8 oz.) package nonfat
cream cheese, softened

3 TB. organic honey

1 cup strawberries, sliced

½ cup kiwi, sliced

¼ cup peaches, pitted
and diced

½ cup blueberries

2 TB. seedless raisins

Each serving has:
220 calories
32 g carbohydrates
9 g fat
3 g fiber
6 g protein

1. Preheat the oven to 375°F.

2. To make pizza crust, combine margarine, ¹/₂ cup sugar, 1 teaspoon cinnamon, 1 teaspoon vanilla, and egg in a medium bowl. Beat until light and fluffy. Add flour and baking powder. Stir well.

3. Spread mixture about ¹/₈-inch thick on a pizza pan or a 9×13-inch baking pan.

4. Bake for 10 to 12 minutes or until lightly golden brown. Cool.

5. To make spread, combine softened cream cheese, 1 tsp. cinnamon, 3 tablespoons honey, and 1 teaspoon vanilla. Spread on cooled pizza crust.

6. Arrange strawberries, kiwi, peaches, blueberries, and raisins on pizza crust. Slice and serve.

Rainbow Crudité Pizza

Yield: 12 servings   *Prep time:* 10 minutes
Cook time: 10 minutes   *Serving size:* 1 slice

16 oz. bread dough, can be bought pre-made

1 cup nonfat sour cream

8 oz. low-calorie cream cheese, softened

¼ tsp. garlic salt

1 (1 oz.) package ranch dressing mix

1 red onion, chopped fine

10 cherry tomatoes, quartered

1 red pepper, chopped

1 green pepper, chopped

1 stalk celery, sliced thin

1 cup broccoli, chopped

1 cup carrot, grated

Each serving has:
195 calories
24 g carbohydrates
5 g fat
3 g fiber
3 g protein

1. Preheat the oven to 350°F degrees. Lightly grease a round 9-inch pan with cooking spray.

2. Press bread dough into bottom of the pan. Bake according to directions on package or follow your own homemade dough recipe. Cool completely.

3. In a large bowl, combine sour cream, cream cheese, garlic salt, and ranch dressing mix. Spread mixture on cooled crust.

4. Place onion, tomatoes, red and green peppers, celery, and broccoli on top cream cheese mixture. Sprinkle with grated carrots. Chill for 3 hours or serve immediately. Caution: do not chill for more than 3 hours or pizza crust will get soggy.

Spinach Fettuccini with Sun Dried Tomatoes and Broccoli Florets

Yield: 6 servings   *Prep time:* 60 minutes
Cook time: 15 minutes   *Serving size:* 1 cup

⅔ cup sun-dried tomato halves, cut into strips

½ cup extra-virgin olive oil

4 cloves garlic, minced

20 oz. frozen chopped broccoli, thawed

Salt and pepper

16 oz. hot, cooked spinach fettuccini

½ cup Parmesan cheese, grated (optional for lower-calorie dish)

Each serving has:
510 calories
80 g carbohydrates
15 g fat
10 g fiber
23 g protein

1. Place sun-dried tomato strips in a bowl. Cover with water. Soften for 1 to 2 hours in the refrigerator. Drain.

2. In a sauté pan over medium-high heat, heat 2 tablespoons olive oil and cook garlic for 3 minutes or until lightly browned.

3. Add remaining olive oil, broccoli, tomatoes, salt, and pepper to the pan. Heat over medium-low heat for 10 minutes or until vegetables are tender.

4. Toss pasta with broccoli sauce. Top with grated Parmesan. Serve.

Colorful Mediterranean Turkey Tortilla Wraps

Yield: 4 servings   *Prep time:* 10 minutes
Cook time: None   *Serving size:* 1 sandwich

4 whole-wheat tortillas, 96 percent fat-free

1 lb. cooked turkey, sliced

1½ cups fresh spinach

1 large red bell pepper, coarsely chopped

1 cup black pitted olives, sliced

1 cup feta cheese

Each serving has:
480 calories
32 g carbohydrates
17 g fat
4 g fiber
40 g protein

1. Lay tortilla flat. To make each wrap, arrange ¼ turkey, ¼ spinach, ¼ red pepper, ¼ cup black olives, and ¼ cup feta cheese on each tortilla wrap.

2. Fold small edge over large edge of wrap. Roll.

3. Midway through wrapping sandwich, fold edges in, to seal. Serve.

Chakra Chili

Yield: 4 servings   *Prep time:* 10 minutes
Cook time: 30 minutes   *Serving size:* 1 cup

2 TB. extra-virgin olive oil

2 large red bell peppers, chopped fine

1 large Vidalia onion, chopped fine

4 cloves garlic, minced

½ tsp. cinnamon

2 tsp. chili powder

2 cups diced tomatoes

½ tsp. salt

1 (15 oz.) can black beans, drained and rinsed

2 cups corn kernels

½ cup low-fat sour cream

Each serving has:
386 calories
65 g carbohydrates
7 g fat
14 g fiber
19 g protein

1. In a large saucepot, heat olive oil over medium-high heat.

2. Sauté peppers for about 5 minutes or until slightly brown and tender. Add onion. Sauté for additional 5 minutes.

3. Add garlic, cinnamon, chili powder, and tomatoes. Cover and simmer for 10 minutes. Add salt, black beans, and corn. Simmer for 15 additional minutes or until heated through.

4. Ladle into portion sizes. Serve each portion with a dollop of fat-free sour cream. Serve.

Black Bean Kaleidoscope Salad

Yield: 6 servings   *Prep time:* 10 minutes
Cook time: 30 minutes   *Serving size:* 1 cup

4 cups black beans, rinsed
and drained

1 cup whole-kernel corn,
frozen (or use fresh)

2 medium tomatoes, seeded
and chopped

¼ cup green onions

¼ cup fresh cilantro

1 medium red onion, diced
fine

2 TB. extra-virgin olive oil

2 TB. lime juice

1 tsp. ground cumin

Salt and pepper

1 cup whole-wheat pasta,
cooked, drained, and
rinsed in cold water

4 cups fresh baby spinach

Each serving has:
498 calories
91 g carbohydrates
7 g fat
21 g fiber
30 g protein

1. In a large bowl, combine black beans, corn, tomatoes, green onions, cilantro, and red onion.

2. In a small bowl, mix olive oil, lime juice, and cumin. Add salt and pepper to taste.

3. Pour contents of the small bowl into the large bowl. Toss well. Add in whole-wheat pasta.

4. Serve mixture on top bed baby spinach.

Exercises to Balance Your Entire Chakra System

In order to maintain your weight loss and a sense of inner peace, it is vital to keep your chakras balanced, as well as your overall lifestyle. The following exercises will help you lead a healthy and peaceful life.

Daily Check-In

One surefire way to ensure that you remain connected to your newfound sense of inner peace is to continue to meditate daily. Before you sit down to meditate, ask yourself the following questions: What is my intention for today? What do I need to learn today? What is my body trying to tell me right now? How can I best serve others and myself today? Simply be still and listen for the answers. When your mind is quiet, you will surely receive the messages you are seeking.

Pay close attention to the coincidences and synchronicities that show up in your life. A famous person once said, "When the student is ready, the teacher will appear." You will be pleasantly astounded at the various teachers that show up in your life, in the form of people, places, and things. Embrace the synchronies, and attempt to remain flexible and open to all the situations you encounter each day.

Pamper Yourself

In order to keep peace and good health flowing into your life, it is vital to nurture yourself on a daily basis. At first, putting your needs ahead of your loved ones may seem extremely selfish and awkward. However, the rewards of caring for yourself will enable you to serve others more fully.

To help others, you must place your own needs and desires first and foremost in your life. At least one day each month, devote one entire day to indulging in yourself. Book a morning at the spa, spend an afternoon at the mall, or leisurely sip a latte at the coffee shop. Although this may seem selfish or unattainable, strive to do it.

Remember that you cannot give away what you do not have. You need to refuel your own tank before giving life energy to others. Find what activities help you refuel and recharge, and engage in them.

Experiment in the Grocery Store

Each time you go to the grocery store, conduct a fun experiment. Find something in the produce aisle that you have never tried before, and bring it home with you. Or take a trip to your local whole-foods store and try a new organic or vegan product that tickles your fancy. Go on an adventure to a vegetable stand that you have never visited before.

Back-to-Nature Journal Exercise

One of the best ways to ground the first chakra and keep all of your energy centers in balance is to spend time outdoors in nature. Nowadays we spend most of our time indoors, sitting in plastic desks under fluorescent lights. As a result, we feel disconnected from life's natural rhythms. In order to thrive, your first chakra needs to be solidly attached to the earth. The best way to root your first chakra to the soil is to learn the secrets Mother Nature has to teach you.

You can acquire this knowledge by observing nature and tapping into its inherent wisdom. An effective way to begin understanding nature's intelligence is to sit outdoors and study an animal indigenous to your area. Squirrels, birds, and rabbits are all excellent creatures to witness in their natural environment. Notice how the squirrel wanders aimlessly from tree to tree, collecting acorns. There appears to be no rhyme or reason to the squirrel's behavior. Watch how the animal collects acorns and then abruptly stops to groom himself or chase another animal friend. Gently pay attention to how the squirrel intently searches for an acorn and quickly scampers away when a nearby bird chirps. The squirrel appears to function quite well without goals, plans, and to-do lists. By relying on his instinct, the squirrel completes all of his daily tasks in perfect order.

Experiment with your own animal instincts this week. Set aside some time to just be, without predetermined goals or ideas about how your time should be spent. During this exercise, pay attention to your own inner drives and intuition. Instead of focusing on outcomes, focus on just being. Listen to your own sense of inner wisdom. After completing this exercise, many people paradoxically report a feeling of increased productivity.

Spend a half-hour outdoors studying nature this week. Answer the following questions in your journal: What did you observe? How did your observations make you feel? What could you accomplish if you relied on your own natural instincts instead of constantly planning, pushing, and making things happen? What have you learned from Mother Nature this week?

Create a Tree Diary

A tree diary is an excellent way to reconnect with nature and reestablish your kinship with Mother Earth. Obtain a blank notebook in which you can create your own tree diary. Ideally, your tree diary should be separate from your journal.

Next, find a tree that you are drawn to and can visit daily. I recommend choosing a tree in your own yard or at a local park that you can visit frequently. Sit down and place your hand on the tree. Feel the energy and life force vibrating through the tree. Notice the sense of electricity that you experience as you handle the branches. Look closely at the leaves and trace its veins with your finger. Either silently or aloud, introduce yourself to the tree and state your intention to learn from the tree.

I realize that this exercise may seem far out and silly at first. Allow yourself to feel awkward and embarrassed. The sense of peace and awe you receive from this exercise will far outweigh your sense of ambivalence. Most people report that this exercise is like revisiting a magical time in childhood. Be sure to write about your experiences in your tree diary.

Day 1: Meditate next to your tree. A good way to establish a relationship with your tree is to meditate next to it. Sit down on the ground next to your tree. Place a pillow underneath you or sit in a chair with both feet placed firmly on the ground if this feels more comfortable to you. Practice the introductory meditation found at the beginning of this chapter, and record your meditation experience in your tree diary.

Day 2: Illustrate your tree. Even if you have not held a crayon since your seventh birthday, you are capable of completing this task. Focus on the process of inventing your own tree portrait. Be playful with your artwork and do not take yourself too seriously.

Day 3: Give a gift to your tree. Today, give thanks to your tree for providing you with oxygen, shade, and beauty. Offer a heartfelt gift to your tree in a way that speaks to you. Your gift can be a prayer, a poem, or an act of service to another person on behalf of the tree. Or you may choose to clean up the backyard or park in which your tree resides.

Day 4: Receive a gift from your tree. Today, receive a gift from your tree. Use your imagination to decide what offering you would most like to receive. Allow the tree to give you the gift of beauty as you enjoy a quiet lunch next to your new friend. Or you may choose to take a fallen leaf from your tree and tape it to one of the pages in your tree diary.

Day 5: Take a photograph of your tree. Today, photograph your tree and place this snapshot in your tree diary. Examine the picture. How does your actual experience of the tree differ from the photograph of the tree? What colors do you see in the photograph? What memories does your tree awaken within you?

Day 6: Make a bark rubbing. Today, bring a piece of paper and crayon outside with you when you visit your tree. Place the paper over the tree's bark and gently press down as you rub the crayon back and forth over the paper. By creating this bark rubbing, you have permanently etched the energy of the tree into the paper. Place the bark rubbing into your tree diary.

Day 7: Plant new life. Today, honor your commitment to nature by creating new life. Plant some new seeds in your backyard or cultivate a vegetable garden. If you do not have access to nature where you live, buy a houseplant or acquire a plot in a communal garden. Or simply write in your tree diary about the beautiful flowers or vegetables that you intend to harvest next season.

In Gratitude

Gratitude is a powerful feeling that emits a high vibrational frequency, eradicating illness and negativity. To experience lasting inner peace, remember to end each day by being grateful for all the gifts in your life. Offer thanks to yourself, your higher power, and those around you on your life's path.

It is helpful to maintain your journal of appreciation and thankfulness. Many people find that the mere practice of keeping a gratitude journal helps them to maintain permanent weight loss.

We would like to conclude this book by thanking you, dear reader, for your time and attention. We are grateful for your support and interest in our work. We wish you peace and love on your journey.

Glossary

accoutrement   An accompaniment, trapping, or garnish.

al dente   Italian for "against the teeth." Refers to pasta or rice that's neither soft nor hard, but just slightly firm against the teeth.

all-purpose flour   Flour that contains only the inner part of the wheat grain. Usable for all purposes from cakes to gravies.

allspice   Named for its flavor of several spices (cinnamon, cloves, nutmeg), allspice is used in many desserts and in rich marinades and stews.

almonds   Mild, sweet, and crunchy nuts that combine nicely with creamy and sweet food items.

amaretto   A popular almond liqueur.

anchovies (also **sardines**)   Tiny, flavorful preserved fish that typically come in cans. Anchovies are a traditional garnish for Caesar salad, the dressing of which contains anchovy paste.

Arborio rice   A plump Italian rice used, among other purposes, for risotto.

artichoke hearts   The center part of the artichoke flower, often found canned in grocery stores.

arugula   A spicy-peppery garden plant with leaves that resemble a dandelion and have a distinctive, sharp flavor.

baby corn   This small version of corn on the cob, eaten whole, is a popular ingredient in Southeast Asian-style cooking.

bake   To cook in a dry oven. Dry-heat cooking often results in a crisping of the exterior of the food being cooked. Moist-heat cooking, through methods such as steaming, poaching, etc., brings a much different, moist quality to the food.

balsamic vinegar   Vinegar produced primarily in Italy from a specific type of grape, which is aged in wood barrels. It is heavier, darker, and sweeter than most vinegars.

bamboo shoots   Crunchy, tasty white parts of the growing bamboo plant, often purchased canned.

barbecue   To quickly cook over high heat, or to cook something long and slow in a rich liquid (barbecue sauce).

basil   A flavorful, almost sweet, resinous herb that is delicious with tomatoes, and used in all kinds of Italian or Mediterranean-style dishes.

beat   To quickly mix substances.

Belgian endive   A plant that resembles a small, elongated, tightly packed head of romaine lettuce. The thick, crunchy leaves can be broken off and used with dips and spreads.

black pepper   A biting and pungent seasoning, freshly ground pepper adds an extra level of flavor and taste to many dishes.

blackening   To cook something quickly in a very hot skillet over high heat, usually with a seasoning mixture. Cajun cooking makes frequent use of blackening.

blanch   To place a food in boiling water for about one minute (or less), to partially cook the exterior and then rinse with cool water to halt the cooking.

blend   To completely mix something, usually with a blender or food processor, more slowly than beating.

bleu cheese   A blue-veined cheese that crumbles easily and has a somewhat soft texture, usually sold in a block. The color is from a flavorful, edible mold that is often added or injected into the cheese.

boil   To heat a liquid to a point where water is forced to turn into steam, causing the liquid to bubble. To boil something is to insert it into boiling water. A rapid boil is when a lot of bubbles form on the surface of the liquid.

bok choy (also **Chinese cabbage**)   A member of the cabbage family with thick stems, crisp texture, and fresh flavor. It's perfect for stir-frying.

bouillon   Dried essence of stock from chicken, beef, vegetable, or other ingredients. This is a popular starting ingredient for soups, as it adds flavor (and often a lot of salt).

breadcrumbs   Tiny pieces of crumbled dry bread, often used for topping or coating.

Brie   A creamy, cow's-milk cheese from France with a soft, edible rind and a mild flavor.

broil   To cook in a dry oven under the overhead high-heat element.

broth   *See* stock.

brown   To cook in a skillet, while turning, until the food's surface is seared and brown in color, to lock in the juices.

brown rice   Whole-grain rice including the germ with a characteristic pale brown or tan color; more nutritious and flavorful than white rice.

bruschetta (or **crostini**)   Slices of toasted or grilled bread with garlic and olive oil, often with other toppings.

bulgur   A wheat kernel that's been steamed, dried, and crushed and is sold in fine and coarse textures.

Cajun cooking   A style of cooking that combines French and Southern characteristics and includes many highly seasoned stews and meats.

capers   Flavorful buds of a Mediterranean plant, ranging in size from a *nonpareil* (about the size of a small pea) to larger, grape-size caper berries.

cappuccino   A coffee drink consisting of equal parts espresso and steamed milk, topped with milk foam.

caramelize   To cook sugar over low heat until it develops a sweet, caramel flavor. The term is increasingly gaining use to describe cooking vegetables (especially onions) or meat in butter or oil over low heat until they soften, sweeten, and develop a caramel color.

caraway   A distinctive, spicy seed used for bread, pork, cheese, and cabbage dishes. It is known to reduce stomach upset, which is why it is often paired with, for example, sauerkraut.

carbohydrate   A nutritional component found in starches, sugars, fruits, and vegetables that causes a rise in blood glucose levels. Carbohydrates supply the body with energy and many important nutrients, including vitamins, minerals, and antioxidants.

cardamom   An intense, sweet-smelling spice, common to Indian cooking, used in baking and coffee.

carob   A tropical tree that produces long pods. The dried, baked, and powdered flesh (carob powder) is used in baking, and the fresh and dried pods are used for a variety of recipes. The flavor is sweet and reminiscent of chocolate.

cayenne   A fiery spice made from hot chile peppers, especially the cayenne chile, a slender, red, and very hot pepper.

cheddar   The ubiquitous, hard, cow's-milk cheese with a rich, buttery flavor that ranges from mellow to sharp. Originally produced in England, cheddar is now produced worldwide.

chiles   Any one of many different "hot" peppers, ranging in intensity from the relatively mild ancho pepper to the blisteringly hot habanero.

chili powder   A seasoning blend that includes chile pepper, cumin, garlic, and oregano. Proportions vary among different versions, but they all offer a warm, rich flavor.

chives   A member of the onion family, chives grow in bunches of long leaves that resemble tall grass or the green tops of onions. They offer a light onion flavor.

chop   To cut into pieces, usually qualified by an adverb such as "*coarsely* chopped," or by a size measurement such as "chopped into 1/2-inch pieces." "Finely chopped" is much closer to mince.

cider vinegar   Vinegar produced from apple cider, popular in North America.

cilantro   A member of the parsley family and used in Mexican cooking (especially salsa) and some Asian dishes. Use in moderation, as the flavor can overwhelm. The seed of the cilantro is the spice coriander.

cinnamon   A sweet, rich, aromatic spice commonly used in baking or desserts. Cinnamon can also be used for delicious and interesting entrées.

clafoutis   A baked, custardlike French dessert and contains fresh fruit.

clove   A sweet, strong, almost wintergreen-flavor spice used in baking and with meats such as ham.

coriander   A rich, warm, spicy seed used in all types of recipes, from African to South American, from entrées to desserts.

count   In terms of seafood or other foods that come in small sizes, the number of that item that compose 1 pound. For example, 31- to 40-count shrimp are large appetizer shrimp often served with cocktail sauce; 51- to 60-count are much smaller.

couscous   Granular semolina (durum wheat) that is cooked and used in many Mediterranean and North African dishes.

crimini mushrooms A relative of the white button mushroom, but it's brown in color and with a richer flavor. The larger, fully grown version is the portobello. *See also* portobello mushrooms.

croutons Chunks of bread, usually between $1/4$- and $1/2$-inch in size, sometimes seasoned and baked, broiled, or fried to a crisp texture. Often used in soups and salads.

crudités Fresh vegetables served as an appetizer, often altogether on one tray.

cumin A fiery, smoky-tasting spice popular in Middle Eastern and Indian dishes. Cumin is a seed; ground cumin seed is the most common form used in cooking.

curry Refers to rich, spicy, Indian-style sauces, and the dishes prepared with them. A curry uses curry powder as its base seasoning.

curry powder A ground blend of rich, flavorful spices used as a basis for curry and many other Indian-influenced dishes. Common ingredients include hot pepper, nutmeg, cumin, cinnamon, pepper, and turmeric. Some curry can also be found in paste form.

custard A cooked mixture of eggs and milk popular as base for desserts.

dash A few drops, usually of a liquid, released by a quick shake, for example, from a bottle of hot sauce.

devein The removal of the dark vein from the back of a large shrimp with a sharp knife.

dice To cut into small cubes about $1/4$-inch square.

Dijon mustard Hearty, spicy mustard made in the style of the Dijon region of France.

dill A herb perfect for eggs, salmon, cheese dishes, and, of course, vegetables (pickles!).

dollop A spoonful of something creamy and thick, like sour cream or whipped cream.

double boiler A set of two pots designed to nest together, one inside the other, and provide consistent, moist heat for foods that need delicate treatment. The bottom pot holds water (not quite touching the bottom of the top pot); the top pot holds the ingredient you want to heat.

dredge   To cover a piece of food with a dry substance such as flour or corn meal.

drizzle   To lightly sprinkle drops of a liquid over food, often as the finishing touch to a dish.

dry   In the context of wine, a wine that contains little or no residual sugar, so it's not very sweet.

entrée   The main dish in a meal. In France, however, the entrée is considered the first course.

extra-virgin olive oil   *See* olive oil.

fennel   In seed form, a fragrant, licorice-tasting herb. The bulbs have a much milder flavor and a celerylike crunch. They are used as a vegetable in salads or cooked recipes.

feta   A white, crumbly, sharp, salty cheese popular in Greek cooking and on salads. Traditional feta is usually made with sheep's milk, but feta-style cheese can be made from sheep's, cow's, or goat's milk.

fillet   A piece of meat or seafood with the bones removed.

flake   To break into thin sections, as with fish.

flaxseed oil   Nutritious oil derived from a blue, flowering plant that contains omega-6 and omega-9 fatty acids, B vitamins, magnesium, lecithin, fiber, protein, and zinc.

floret   The flower or bud end of broccoli or cauliflower.

flour   Grains ground into a meal. Wheat is perhaps the most common flour. Flour is also made from oats, rye, buckwheat, soybeans, etc. *See also* all-purpose flour; cake flour; whole-wheat flour.

fold   To combine a dense and light mixture with a circular action from the middle of the bowl.

frittata   A skillet-cooked mixture of eggs and other ingredients that's not stirred but is cooked slowly; it's then either flipped or finished under the broiler.

fry   *See* sauté.

garbanzo beans (or **chickpeas**)   A yellow-gold, roundish bean used as the base ingredient in hummus. Chickpeas are high in fiber and low in fat.

garlic A member of the onion family, a pungent and flavorful element in many savory dishes. A garlic bulb contains multiple cloves. Each clove, when chopped, provides about 1 teaspoon garlic. Most recipes call for cloves or chopped garlic by the teaspoon.

garnish An embellishment not vital to the dish but added to enhance visual appeal.

ginger Available in fresh root or dried, ground form, ginger adds a pungent, sweet, and spicy quality to a dish.

Gorgonzola A creamy, rich Italian bleu cheese. *Dolce* is sweet, and that's the kind you want.

grate To shave into tiny pieces using a sharp rasp or grater.

grind To reduce a large, hard substance to the consistency of sand. Often done with a seasoning such as peppercorns.

handful An unscientific measurement; the amount of an ingredient you can hold in your hand.

hazelnuts (also **filberts**) A sweet nut popular in desserts and, to a lesser degree, in savory dishes.

hoisin sauce A sweet Asian condiment similar to ketchup, made with soybeans, sesame, chile peppers, and sugar.

hors d'oeuvre French for "outside of work" (the "work" being the main meal), an hors d'oeuvre can be any dish served as a starter before the meal.

horseradish A sharp, spicy root that forms the flavor base in many condiments from cocktail sauce to sharp mustards. Prepared horseradish contains vinegar and oil, among other ingredients. Use pure horseradish much more sparingly than the prepared version, or try cutting it with sour cream.

hummus A thick, Middle Eastern spread made of puréed garbanzo beans, lemon juice, olive oil, garlic, and often tahini (sesame seed paste).

infusion A liquid in which flavorful ingredients such as herbs have been soaked or steeped to extract that flavor into the liquid.

Italian seasoning A blend of dried herbs, including basil, oregano, rosemary, and thyme.

jicama A juicy, crunchy, sweet, large, round Central American vegetable. If you can't find jicama, try substituting sliced water chestnuts.

julienne   A French word meaning "to slice into very thin pieces."

kalamata olives   Traditionally from Greece, these medium-small, long, black olives have a smoky, rich flavor.

knead   To work dough to make it pliable, so that it holds gas bubbles as it bakes. Kneading is fundamental in the process of making yeast breads.

kosher salt   A coarse-grained salt made without any additives or iodine.

lentils   Tiny lens-shaped pulses used in European, Middle Eastern, and Indian cuisines.

marinate   To soak meat, seafood, or other food in a seasoned sauce, called a marinade, which is high in acid content. The acids break down the muscle of the meat, making it tender and adding flavor.

marjoram   A sweet herb, a cousin of and similar to oregano, popular in Greek, Spanish, and Italian dishes.

meld   To allow flavors to blend and spread over time. Melding is often why recipes call for overnight refrigeration; it is also why some dishes taste better as leftovers.

meringue   A baked mixture of sugar and beaten egg whites, often used as a dessert topping.

mesclun   Mixed salad greens, usually containing lettuce and assorted greens such as arugula, cress, endive, and others.

mince   To cut into very small pieces, smaller than diced pieces, about 1/8 inch or smaller.

miso   A fermented, flavorful soybean paste, key in many Japanese dishes.

mold   A decorative, shaped metal pan in which contents, such as mousse or gelatin, set up and take the shape of the pan.

nutmeg   A sweet, fragrant, musky spice used primarily in baking.

olive oil   A fragrant oil produced by crushing or pressing olives. Extra-virgin olive oil—the most flavorful and highest quality—is produced from the first pressing of a batch of olives; oil is also produced from later pressings.

olives   The fruit of the olive tree commonly grown on all sides of the Mediterranean. Black olives are also called ripe olives. Green olives are immature, although they are also widely eaten. *See also* kalamata olives.

oregano A fragrant, slightly astringent herb used in Greek, Spanish, and Italian dishes.

orzo A rice-shaped pasta used in Greek cooking.

oxidation The browning of fruit flesh that happens over time and with exposure to air. Minimize oxidation by rubbing the cut surfaces with a lemon half. Oxidation also affects wine, which is why the taste changes over time after a bottle is opened.

paprika A rich, red, warm, earthy spice that also lends a rich, red color to many dishes.

Parmesan A hard, dry, flavorful cheese primarily used grated or shredded as a seasoning for Italian-style dishes.

parsley A fresh-tasting, green, leafy herb, often used as a garnish.

pecans Rich, buttery nuts, native to North America, that have a high unsaturated-fat content.

pesto A thick spread or sauce made with fresh basil leaves, garlic, olive oil, pine nuts, and Parmesan cheese. Some newer versions are made with other herbs.

pickle A food, usually a vegetable such as a cucumber, that's been pickled in brine.

pinch An unscientific measurement term, the amount of an ingredient—typically a dry, granular substance such as an herb or seasoning—you can hold between your finger and thumb.

pita bread A hollow, flat wheat bread often used in slices for sandwiches or topped pizza-style. Soft, baked, or broiled, it's terrific with dips or as a vehicle for other ingredients.

plantain A relative of the banana, a plantain is larger, milder in flavor, and used as a staple in many Latin American dishes.

porcini mushrooms Rich, flavorful mushrooms used in rice and Italian-style dishes.

portobello mushrooms A mature and larger form of the smaller crimini mushroom, portobellos are brownish, chewy, and flavorful. Often served as whole caps, grilled, and as thin sautéed slices. *See also* crimini mushrooms.

preheat   To turn on an oven, broiler, or other cooking appliance in advance of cooking so the temperature will be at the desired level when the assembled dish is ready for cooking.

purée   To reduce a food to a thick, creamy texture, usually by using a blender or food processor.

reduce   To boil or simmer a broth or sauce to remove some of the water content, resulting in more concentrated flavor and color.

reserve   To hold a specified ingredient for another use, later in the recipe.

rice vinegar   Vinegar produced from fermented rice or rice wine, popular in Asian-style dishes. Different from rice wine vinegar.

ricotta   A fresh Italian cheese smoother than cottage cheese with a slightly sweet flavor.

risotto   A popular Italian rice dish made by browning Arborio rice in butter or oil, and then slowly adding liquid to cook the rice, resulting in a creamy texture.

roast   To cook something uncovered in an oven, usually without additional liquid.

rosemary   A pungent, sweet herb used with chicken, pork, fish, and especially lamb. A little of it goes a long way.

saffron   A spice made from the stamens of crocus flowers, saffron lends a dramatic yellow color and distinctive flavor to a dish. Use only tiny amounts of this expensive herb.

sage   An herb with a musty yet fruity, lemon-rind scent and "sunny" flavor.

salsa   A style of mixing fresh vegetables and/or fresh fruit in a coarse chop. Salsa can be spicy or not, fruit-based or not, and served as a starter on its own (with chips, for example) or as a companion to a main course.

sauté   To pan-cook over lower heat than used for frying.

savory   A popular herb with a fresh, woody taste.

sear   To quickly brown the exterior of a food, especially meat, over high heat, to preserve interior moisture.

Serrano pepper A type of chili pepper that originated in the Mexican states of Puebla and Hildago. These peppers can be green, brown, red, orange, or yellow in color and are typically between 1 to 3 inches long.

sesame oil An oil, made from pressing sesame seeds, that's tasteless if clear, and is aromatic and flavorful if brown.

shallot A member of the onion family that grows in a bulb somewhat like garlic, and has a milder onion flavor. When a recipe calls for shallot, use the entire bulb.

shellfish A broad range of seafood, including clams, mussels, oysters, crabs, shrimp, and lobster. Some people are allergic to shellfish, so take care with its inclusion in recipes.

shiitake mushrooms Large, dark brown mushrooms with a hearty, meaty flavor. Can be used either fresh or dried, grilled, or as a component in other recipes, and as a flavoring source for broth.

shred To cut into many long, thin slices.

short-grain rice A starchy rice, popular for Asian-style dishes because it readily clumps (perfect for eating with chopsticks).

simmer To boil gently so the liquid barely bubbles.

skewers Thin wooden or metal sticks, usually about 8 inches long, used for assembling kebabs, dipping food pieces into hot sauces, or serving single-bite food items with a bit of panache.

skillet (also **frying pan**) A generally heavy, flat-bottomed metal pan with a handle, designed to cook food over heat on a stovetop or campfire.

skim To remove fat or other material from the top of liquid.

slice To cut into thin pieces.

steam To suspend a food over boiling water and allow the heat of the steam (water vapor) to cook the food. A quick-cooking method, steaming preserves the flavor and texture of a food.

stew To slowly cook pieces of food submerged in a liquid. Also refers to a dish that has been prepared by this method.

stir-fry To cook small pieces of food in a wok or skillet over high heat, moving and turning the food quickly to cook all sides.

stock   A flavorful broth made by cooking meats and/or vegetables with seasonings until the liquid absorbs these flavors. This liquid is then strained, and the solids discarded. Can be eaten alone or used as a base for soups, stews, etc.

tahini   A paste made from sesame seeds, and used to flavor many Middle Eastern recipes.

tarragon   A sweet, rich-smelling herb perfect with seafood, vegetables (especially asparagus), chicken, and pork.

teriyaki   A Japanese-style sauce composed of soy sauce, rice wine, ginger, and sugar that works well with seafood as well as most meats.

thyme   A minty, zesty herb.

toast   To heat something, usually bread, so it's browned and crisp.

tofu   A cheeselike substance made from soybeans and soy milk.

tomatillo   A small, round fruit with a distinctive, spicy flavor, often found in south-of-the-border dishes. To use, remove the papery outer skin, rinse off any sticky residue, and chop like a tomato.

turmeric   A spicy, pungent, yellow root used in many dishes, especially Indian cuisine, for color and flavor. Turmeric is the source of the yellow color in many prepared mustards.

twist   A garnish for an appetizer or other dish, usually made from a lemon or other citrus fruit. To make, cut a thin, $^{1}/_{8}$-inch-thick cross-section slice of a lemon or other fruit. Cut from the center of that slice, out to the edge on one side. Pull apart the two cut ends in opposite directions.

vinegar   An acidic liquid widely used as dressing and seasoning, often made from fermented grapes, apples, or rice. *See also* balsamic vinegar; cider vinegar; rice vinegar; white vinegar; wine vinegar.

walnuts   A rich, slightly wood-flavored nut.

wasabi   Japanese horseradish, a fiery, pungent condiment used with many Japanese-style dishes. Most often sold as a powder, and then water added to create a paste.

water chestnuts   A tuber, popular in many types of Asian-style cooking. The flesh is white, crunchy, and juicy, and the vegetable holds its texture whether cool or hot.

whisk To rapidly mix, introducing air to the mixture.

white mushrooms Button mushrooms. When fresh, they have an earthy smell and an appealing "soft crunch."

white vinegar The most common type of vinegar, produced from grain.

whole-wheat flour Wheat flour that contains the entire grain.

wine vinegar Vinegar produced from red or white wine.

wok A pan for quick-cooking.

yeast Tiny fungi that, when mixed with water, sugar, flour, and heat, release carbon dioxide bubbles, which in turn, cause the bread to rise.

zest Small slivers of peel, usually from a citrus fruit such as lemon, lime, or orange.

Index

M